Lose Weight

Without Dieting or Working Out!

ALSO BY JJ SMITH

10-Day Green Smoothie Cleanse

Lose Weight

Without Dieting or Working Out!

JJ Smith

ATRIA PAPERBACK

NEW YORK   LONDON   TORONTO   SYDNEY   NEW DELHI

ATRIA PAPERBACK

Atria Paperback
A Division of Simon & Schuster, Inc.
1230 Avenue of the Americas
New York, NY 10020

Copyright © 2012, 2013 by Jennifer (JJ) Smith
This work was previously self-published.

First Atria Paperback edition July 2014

ATRIA PAPERBACK and colophon are trademarks of Simon & Schuster, Inc.

For information about special discounts for bulk purchases, please contact Simon & Schuster Special Sales at 1-866-506-1949 or business@simonandschuster.com.

The Simon & Schuster Speakers Bureau can bring authors to your live event. For more information or to book an event, contact the Simon & Schuster Speakers Bureau at 1-866-248-3049 or visit our website at www.simonspeakers.com.

Manufactured in the United States of America

10 9 8 7 6 5 4 3 2 1

Library of Congress Cataloging-in-Publication Data is available.

ISBN 978-1-4767-9999-5
ISBN 978-1-5011-0009-3 (ebook)

Contents

Important Note to Readers

The information contained in this book is for your education. It is not intended to diagnose, treat, or cure any medical condition or dispense medical advice. If you decide to follow my plan, you should seek the advice and counsel of your licensed health professional and then use your own judgment.

It is important to obtain proper medical advice before you make any decisions about nutrition, diet, supplements, or other health-related issues that are discussed in this book. Neither the author nor the publisher is qualified to provide medical, financial, or psychological advice or services. The reader should consult an appropriate healthcare professional before heeding any of the advice given in this book.

Preface

I am a nutritionist and certified weight-management expert who has seen firsthand that *what you eat* is the most crucial aspect of managing weight and is much more important than traditional dieting or exercising. I wrote this book because I made a personal commitment to help others get slimmer, sexier, and healthier. My goal is to give you all the information you need to lose weight and get healthy. I will provide you with the knowledge, skills, and guidelines that you can use in your life to not only lose weight but also to restore your health and energy.

When I was in my twenties, I could eat anything I wanted and still stay slim. Unfortunately, I practiced poor eating habits. I was a junk-food and fast-food junkie. When I was in my thirties, my health began to deteriorate, and as my metabolism slowed, my weight began to increase. I eventually gained forty pounds and went up four dress sizes. However, of even greater concern were the numerous health ailments and illnesses that I began to experience.

I tried many popular diets, but they required too much discipline and only worked as long as I stayed on them. But who wants to be on a diet all the time? I learned that if you go on a diet, at some point, when you go off the diet, you typically gain the weight back. While you're on it, you starve and crave foods, and as soon as you go off it, you eat all the foods that caused you to gain weight in the first place. In order to be successful, you have to break the addiction to foods that cause you to gain weight. If you crave them, you will always fail on a diet...until the addiction is broken once and for all. So, I got off diets and changed my lifestyle to lose weight, regain energy, and restore my health.

At one point, when I was in my twenties, my doctors gave me antibiotics that I took every day for several months to cure acne. Years later, I found out that this lengthy period of medication had taken a toll on the internal balance in my system: I had an overgrowth of intestinal bacteria and was diagnosed with candidiasis. Furthermore, for years, I kept getting sick with numerous ailments and illnesses. I was diagnosed with sinus infections, yeast infections, arthritis, chronic fatigue, prediabetes/insulin resistance, hernias, polyps, and ovarian cysts. Many of these conditions required surgery. Sometimes, I just felt generally rundown and exhausted, having little to no energy. I became frustrated! The doctors' answers were not getting me well. So I researched everything I could about different ways to heal my body and get healthy. The more techniques I tried, the better I started to look and feel. In fact, something very interesting happened. The more I applied natural practices of healing, the more I slimmed down and the more youthful I began to look. It was as though I was turning back the hands of time. At that point, I knew I was on the right path toward staying slim and healthy and getting my life back!

By the time I was in my late thirties, I had really started to heavily research, study, and apply knowledge about how to heal my body and lose weight. I learned the science of how the body responds to different foods, how hormones play a role in weight gain, and how to speed up my metabolism to reverse the natural slowing of metabolism that happens as we age. I began to get amazing results. I even went on to receive several certifications—one as a certified nutritionist and another as a certified weight-management expert. Now, in my forties, I teach my numerous clients these techniques to stay slim, restore health, and get their sexy back!

I realized that by adopting a healthy diet and lifestyle—one that involved regular internal cleansing and detoxification—I could regain control of my body and my well-being. Since then, it has become my passion to educate others and share with them the natural remedies that helped me achieve the superb health that I enjoy today. I have dedicated my life to the field of healthy eating and living. I have studied many philosophies of health and natural healing and learned from some of the great teachers of our time.

Today, while many women over forty have concerns about their changing shape, I've been able to keep my body pretty fat-resistant, even now that I am in my forties and dealing with perimenopause. I discovered an entirely new approach to managing my weight that is designed to address the real underlying causes of weight gain. It is so much more complicated than eating less and exercising more. In this book, I address the real reasons we become overweight or obese. Most diet plans address only one or two of these factors; my system—which I call the DEM System—addresses all of them.

I firmly believe that every individual person is responsible for his or her own health and wellness. If you want to be healthy and energetic and look vibrant, you must learn what is involved and apply it to your life. You have to watch what goes into your mouth, how much physical activity you get, and what thoughts you think. You need to cleanse and detoxify your body and eat "clean and balanced" foods that provide nutrients that fuel your body throughout the day. I make the commitment to staying on top of this valuable information every day. The good news is that you can, too! It is very easy because this knowledge is readily available to you. Of course, health professionals can give you valuable information and help you treat illness and diseases, but in the end, the responsibility rests on your shoulders.

Thousands of studies support the foundational principles of the DEM System you are about to learn. And I have personally seen the techniques work for myself and for thousands of people who have achieved optimal health and vitality. I have applied these principles for more than ten years and currently conduct teleseminars guiding people through the experience you are about to embark on. The results that are possible within a few short weeks are remarkable.

You, too, can now take advantage of the DEM System I have developed to help you achieve quick and sustainable weight loss and begin a new lifestyle of healthy eating and living. It's time to stop dieting and start living!

Introduction

Battling excess weight can be one of the most frustrating, challenging, and emotionally draining experiences on earth. Despite the numerous diets, exercise regimens, and magic pills for weight loss, Americans continue to grow larger and larger year after year. More than two thirds of the adult population and one third of our children are now overweight. Obesity rates have tripled since the 1960s.

Diets abound, and the diet industry is huge. But the sad fact is that about 95 percent of people who lose weight on a diet gain the weight back in three to five years. You cannot lose weight permanently by strictly following any special diet, by taking a weight-loss pill, or by following an exercise regimen.

The good news is that anyone can lose weight and stay slim if he or she just understands, addresses, and corrects the hidden causes of weight gain. In order to succeed in the battle of the bulge, you have to realize that losing weight involves a major lifestyle change.

To ensure you understand what I mean by "lifestyle change," I want to take a moment to explain this further. As the title *Lose Weight Without Dieting or Working Out* implies, you have to do two things to ensure that you achieve a "lifestyle change." First, you will have to forget about dieting! Typically, you "go on" a diet, which implies that at some point you "go off" the diet. A typical diet is something you do for a specified period of time. However, what usually happens when you "go off" the diet? You gain all the weight back. So, we are going to retrain your taste buds to desire and crave healthier foods so you never have to think about dieting again. Chapter 1 explains why dieting is not the most effective way to lose weight permanently. Second, you don't have to stress about maintaining a rigorous exercise routine to lose weight. As Chapter 2 explains, studies show why intense exercise or working out is not critical for weight loss. Instead, we're going to teach you how to simply "get moving" by being more physically active throughout the day, even if you don't get to a gym to "work out." As the title implies, from this point forward, you can actually forget about dieting and stop stressing about working out and get ready for a true "lifestyle change."

The goal of my book is simple: to show you how to lose weight *permanently* and achieve optimal health. You can achieve this without counting calories or measuring portion sizes or eating bland, packaged foods. Instead, you will enjoy fresh, delicious, healthy foods that will nourish every cell in your body so that you not only get slim, but healthy and vibrant as well. Your skin will become brighter, your eyes will sparkle, your hair will get shinier, and your overall look will be radiant and beautiful!

The information in this book is different from that of any other diet or detox book. It is a combination of information that I have learned as a certified nutritionist and certified weight-management expert. I've acquired this knowledge from many different teachers, health practitioners, training programs, mentors, and friends. These concepts are based on sound research and the work of many doctors, scientists, and research institutions. Some of the topics I'll discuss still have not made it into mainstream health and nutrition practices. However, the good news is that all my research, study, and practical application have paid off for me and my numerous clients, who have lost weight and kept it off!

This book explains the strongest, most-compelling, and best-supported principles of permanent weight loss that anyone can follow, no matter their size, income level, or educational level. And the end result is a sexy, healthy, beautiful body. If you have been on a rollercoaster ride of weight loss, you will finally be able to get off and achieve your healthy, ideal weight.

This book is for you if you are sick, tired, overweight, and frustrated; you've lost weight and gained it all back; you diet and exercise, yet the weight never seems to melt away. Have you tried:

- Counting calories or points throughout the day?
- Using your willpower to resist sweets and junk food?
- Working out in the gym like a maniac four to five times a week?
- Cutting fats and carbs and measuring portion sizes of everything you eat?

Traditional dieting is sheer torture and costly, with results being hit or miss. I've been there. You have to suppress cravings, eat foods that taste boring, and feel continually hungry, only to regain the weight after the diet ends. If you have tried any of the traditional dieting approaches with little to no success, you are not alone. They simply are not effective for losing weight permanently.

Some of you may have picked up this book to shed a few pounds for a special occasion, while others may have a more significant amount of weight to lose. Some of you have found that taking weight off is relatively easy but keeping it off long term is a lifelong challenge. Maybe you have simply been single too long and want to make a concerted attempt to look more attractive to the opposite sex. Maybe you're a parent trying to help your overweight child gain control of his or her eating habits. There is no bad reason to begin on this journey to lose weight, heal your body, and regain a second youth.

The Detox, Eat, Move (DEM) System

The DEM System is a breakthrough permanent weight-loss solution that melts fat from your body, especially from stubborn areas like the hips, thighs, and belly, through detoxifying and cleansing the body and feeding it healthy, nutrient-rich foods that keep it slim. Even if obesity runs in your family, you can break that hereditary cycle with this new approach to managing your weight. You can't change your genes, but by simply eating smart, you can manage how your body functions to optimize your health.

The DEM System achieves far more than what traditional dieting accomplishes. It is a complete weight-management program designed to help your body clear out old toxic waste that contributes to excess fat in the body. By following the DEM System, you can learn what many people don't know and what celebrities pay thousands of dollars to famous doctors to learn. You will learn about how your body responds to certain foods, how to achieve excellent health, and how to maintain a healthy, ideal weight.

With the DEM System, you will never count calories or have to follow complicated and expensive meal plans or measure food again. After the initial detoxification phase of the DEM System, you will not only eat well, you also will begin to desire healthy, natural foods.

And here's my favorite part of the DEM System: you will see results even if you don't maintain an exercise regimen. If you already exercise, then, of course, you will accelerate your progress and gain the great benefits of exercising. Since we all know that physical activity is good for general health, I will provide some simple ways to "get moving" without having to go somewhere (like to a gym) to get your workout on. However, even if you don't exercise, you will still see results.

For those who think I'm going to tell you to work out in a gym three to four times per week, you're in for a pleasant surprise. You can reach your ideal weight without any formal exercise regimen when you follow the DEM System. You will also enjoy generous amounts of tasty, satisfying foods. I believe food is to be enjoyed and should help us not only maintain great health, but also help us stay slim and lean.

Following the DEM System, you will give your body the quality nutrition it needs while cleansing your cells on an ongoing basis. Vitamins, minerals, and other nutrients will be absorbed by your body more efficiently, allowing your cells to become like new as you begin to look and feel younger. Your skin will begin to look more youthful because your cells become tighter and healthier. Aging, dull, dry skin; puffiness; dark circles; and wrinkles will start to fade away. It is possible to look and feel better now than you did a decade ago. You will feel like you're growing younger, not older! What makes us feel old is sludge and waste in the body. Even if you opt for anti-aging creams and cosmetic surgery, you cannot fully slow the aging process without cleaning out the sludge and waste in your body. In short, you'll learn how to become young, healthy, and energetic from the inside out.

I'm not going to tell you that the DEM System is simple and easy. The fact of the matter is that the first twenty-one days will be the hardest part but also the most rewarding, as it tends to result in rapid weight loss (fat loss). You will also reprogram your body to continue to lose weight until you get your desired "naturally thin" body. You will eat nutritious, healthy foods and stop eating unhealthy junk foods that cause weight gain and provide no nutritional value. I will help you train your body to enjoy vegetables, lean meat, fruits, nuts, and seeds and to shun the unhealthy crap. I will ask you to cut out fatty, sugary junk foods and to simply "get moving" without going to the gym.

I will often discuss strategies for "losing weight," but in reality, what you want to lose is fat; you actually want to shrink fat cells in the body. The focus isn't going to be on the number on the scale as much as on the loss of body fat and inches.

Even if you have given up on losing weight due to your age and hectic lifestyle, you can lose excess body fat very quickly on this program. You can achieve a lean, healthy body for life.

What's in this Book?

The strategies presented in this book will provide greater long-term success than any other diet or exercise program you may have tried in the past. This book addresses all of the underlying causes of weight gain and poor health in a comprehensive system that will result in permanent weight loss. You will lose body fat and see a decrease in your clothing size all while watching your overall health and happiness levels increase to a level you may have never thought possible.

In Part 1, I discuss what makes most people overweight and unhealthy. This will help you understand what has been going on in your body causing you to gain weight. You'll come to understand why you crave certain foods and learn what types of foods cause fat to melt away. We begin by debunking many of the misconceptions about weight loss. You will discover how much of what you have learned about dieting is wrong, ineffective, or unhealthy.

In Part 2, I give you the keys to turning your body into a fat-burning machine that allows your body to lose weight effortlessly. You'll learn the techniques and methods to sculpt a fat-burning body without strenuous exercise. You'll gain a practical understanding of the principles behind permanent weight loss, which include getting rid of toxins, balancing your hormones, and speeding up your metabolism. You will also learn which foods help you stay slim and which cause you to get fat.

In Part 3, I detail the DEM System to guide you along each step of your weight-loss plan. You will learn how to detoxify the body, eat "clean and balanced" foods, and get moving without "working out." I will provide you with a wealth of information, including a detailed list of delicious foods, supplements, and other detox methods to support you through the program. You'll be surprised to find that your body will begin to crave healthy foods, allowing you to easily follow this program. All you'll need to do is follow the guidelines in each phase of the program and listen to your body, which will repay you with the shedding of pounds as it savors the many delicious food choices. I believe it is more effective than any other weight-loss program available today.

In Part 4, I speak directly about the weight issues affecting women. I discuss how to achieve great health, beauty, and vibrancy. I'll discuss problem areas for women over forty who are fighting aging skin, wrinkles, cellulite, and belly fat—as well as that unexplained weight gain that occurs during perimenopause and menopause—and fun and sexy ways to get fit without traditional exercise. I'll also help you regain your self-confidence and self-esteem to keep you motivated throughout the program.

Your Weight Loss Journey Begins Today!

My goal is to make you, my reader, understand that you can avoid wasting time and energy on traditional diets that only provide temporary weight loss. Know that you can achieve your most beautiful self and your perfect weight while still eating abundantly. When you are no longer worrying about your weight, you can focus on your life dreams and goals.

Keep in mind that you are an individual, which means your journey to weight loss will be uniquely personal to you. You will discover what techniques work well for you, what roadblocks you may need to overcome, and, most importantly, how to encourage and motivate yourself. I've tried to explain the steps in the DEM System as clearly as possible so the dietary and lifestyle changes ensure steady and consistent progress and don't make you feel overwhelmed. The DEM System is your personal journey toward your weight-loss destination.

I suggest you read this book just for understanding at first and then reread it with a mind to take action and begin your journey. Get a copy for a family member and friend so that you all can encourage and support one another through this life-changing transformation. Your family, friends, and I will be here to guide you along and support you. I have had frustrations with unexplained weight gain. I have worked hard to lose weight, only to find that each week, the pounds continued to pile on. You are not alone. We will do this together. Let your journey begin today.

Lastly, I want to congratulate you for having the courage to take back control of your weight and your health. We are surrounded by so many unhealthy food choices that are enticing and addictive. But with the proper guidance and motivation, you can leave old eating habits behind and establish new, healthier eating habits. Know that this will take resolve, discipline, and the ability to overcome short-term temptation, but those temptations will diminish significantly after the first month of the DEM System. I know how much courage it takes to begin a new life and a new relationship with food. I support you and encourage you in your efforts.

Sincerely,

JJ Smith

PART 1

What Makes Us Overweight and Unhealthy?

What Makes Us
Overweight and Unhealthy?

I believe that most overweight people are actually natural-ly thin. The body is complex and designed to maintain healthiness. The body is smarter than any diet pill or fad diet on the market. If you just change your eating habits to align with your body's natural ability to heal, stay slim, and have energy, you will never have to worry about weight again. So, in this book, we are going to change the way you think about weight loss and eating forever.

People who do not struggle with weight problems seem to think the cause of obesity is simply laziness and gluttony. In fact, I really get tired of people assuming that overweight or obese people should just eat less and exercise more to lose weight. This is an overly simplistic view of the problem. The mantra of "eat less and exercise more" does not solve the many complicated factors affecting weight gain for most people. You need to understand that the human body is much more complex than this as it relates to weight loss. I've heard everything from "stop eating so much" and "step away from the table" to "overweight peo-ple are lazy and have no willpower." It's a false message to send to overweight people that being fat is totally their fault. This is simply not true. We may have heard an over-weight person say, "I don't really eat that much, and I still can't seem to lose weight." Often they are telling the truth. In fact, I think we all know people who are overweight who work very hard to lose weight to no avail. They count calories, eat less, and work out but get little in the way of long-term or permanent results.

The truth is that nobody wants to be fat. Excess weight is due to a combination of factors that are often outside of one's control, such as genetics, hormonal imbalances, or the poor-quality Standard American Diet (SAD) readily available to us. It isn't your fault that you have problems with your weight. Even if you have enough willpower to keep yourself from eating when your brain tells you that you're hungry, you still may not be able to lose weight. There are so many other factors in play that cause you to gain weight. Until you understand the real reasons you gain weight, you will never be able to lose weight permanently. The key is to learn to naturally speed up your body's fat-burning capabilities to help you lose weight and get healthy.

There is no one simple reason why an individual may have trouble with his or her weight; in most cases, there are several reasons. I will share all of them with you so you can understand how to assist your own body in becoming naturally thin and healthy.

CHAPTER ONE

Why Diets Fail You

Diets are not the most effective way to lose weight permanently. Your goal should be to change your lifestyle, including proper nutrition and getting physically active, as a way to achieve your weight-loss goals. When most people think of dieting, they immediately think of eating less, which is a flawed dieting technique that allows you to lose weight in the short term but rarely allows you to keep the weight off permanently.

Even if you achieve your weight-loss goals through a particular diet, you will slowly gain the weight right back. The problem is that you "go on" a diet, which implies that you also later "go off" the diet. A typical diet is something you do for a short period of time. Therein lies the reason 95 percent of people who lose weight on a diet gain it back. In fact, if someone tells me they've lost twenty or thirty pounds on some great new diet, I tell them to come back in six months' time. If they have maintained their weight loss, then I'm willing to listen about this great new diet. By then, in many cases, they have unfortunately already begun to gain all the weight back.

Too many diets force you to eat bland, prepackaged, unappetizing food or chalky-tasting milkshakes. This causes you to crave and fantasize about all the delicious foods you can't have on your diet. These cravings or mental images challenge your willpower and cause you to give in to the foods you're missing, making you feel like you've failed on your diet again. My plan allows you to discover whole, natural foods that are healthy and palatable, without the empty calories.

The beauty of fresh, whole foods is that you can eat them abundantly and still lose weight. When you eat high-sugar/high-fat foods, you tend to keep on eating and eating because sugar and fat don't make us feel full and cause us to crave more sugar and fat. However, whole, natural foods (fruits, veggies, whole grains) are nutrient-rich, high in fiber, and make us feel full and satisfied so we don't overeat.

Diets require that you eat less and lower your calorie intake, but if you don't provide your body with adequate nutrition, it will go into starvation mode and begin to hold on to fat for future use. Fat cells respond to starvation by holding on to the fat they already have as a survival mechanism, making it more difficult to shed fat in the long run. However, if you give your body the proper nutrition, it will shed fat, and the pounds will melt away without you even making an effort. When we consistently provide the body with good nutrition, the brain no longer believes the body is dieting, so it "relaxes" and stops telling the body to hold on to fat. As an example, if you skip breakfast to cut calories and lose weight, your stomach will begin to growl and send a message to your brain that you are starving, and it will immediately begin to store fat for future use in case your body does not receive any more food.

Any diet that deprives us of nutrients works against

our weight-loss efforts. Even if you decide to lower your caloric intake, you still must be sure to eat high-quality foods that contain a lot of nutrients and vitamins. This is the key to losing weight.

Why Calorie-Counting Is Useless

Most diets focus on restricting calories partly by cutting back on the amount of food eaten. But calorie restriction doesn't work in and of itself; losing weight is not just about eating less. In fact, if you eat too little, you set off a chain of chemical imbalances in your hormones and brain that actually cause you to gain weight.

Yes, calories are important. But it is not the *number* of calories you consume as much as it is the *type* of calories that makes all the difference between how much weight you lose and how healthy you are.

You can actually have an identical amount of calories from sugary foods (cupcake) and lean proteins (turkey breast), but the metabolic effect will be entirely different. The nutrients in sugary foods are different from the nutrients in lean proteins, and so they cause a different hormonal response, which plays a key role in determining what happens to those calories, such as how much of them end up being stored as fat in the body. This is why calorie counting simply does not work for weight loss.

What is a calorie? A calorie is simply a unit of energy. A more scientific definition states it as the quantity of energy required to raise the temperature of one gram of water by one degree Celsius under standard conditions. Simply stated, calories are units of energy that fuel our bodies, just as gasoline fuels our cars. We get calories from the food we eat. When we consume food, our body breaks down this food and turns it into energy. We consume calories so that we will have something to burn. The average adult body needs at least 1,000 to 1,400 calories to have enough energy to fuel key organs like the heart, brain, and lungs—to keep the basic functions of our body operating. This minimum number of calories is called your resting metabolic rate (RMR) and it varies depending upon your sex, age, weight, and muscle mass. You then need some additional calories (400 to 600) just to move and be active throughout the day. When you severely restrict caloric intake, it causes the number of calories you consume to drop below your resting metabolic rate. This then falls below the basic amount of energy or calories you need to fuel your body for the day.

The commonly stated logic is that if you eat the same number of calories you burn, you will stay the same weight. If you eat less than you burn, you will lose weight; if you eat more calories than you burn, you will gain weight. This seems to make sense, but it does not tell the whole story. As an example, let's look at the difference between 1,000 calories of lima beans versus 1,000 calories of a low-fat cinnamon raisin bagel. As far as calories go, they are both 1,000 calories. But because each item has a different amount of protein, fat, carbs, and fiber, the nutrients are absorbed into the body at different rates, sending different metabolic signals that ultimately control your weight. The carbs (sugar) from the lima beans enter your bloodstream very slowly, but the carbs from the low-fat cinnamon raisin bagel enter your bloodstream very rapidly. The calories from the lima beans will be absorbed over time and thus used over a longer period of time for energy. However, the calories from the cinnamon raisin bagel go into your bloodstream all at once, and any calories that can't be used right away for energy will get stored as fat. This mean the low-fat cinnamon raisin bagel causes more fat storage in the body, even though it has the same number of calories as the lima beans. Here's the general rule of thumb: foods whose calories enter your bloodstream quickly promote weight gain, whereas foods whose calories enter your bloodstream slowly promote weight loss. So, you can see why calorie-counting alone is not effective for managing weight loss.

We are not going to be counting calories in the DEM System. I never count calories. For generations, people stayed slim and healthy without ever counting calories. Decades ago, people weren't focused on counting calories to stay slim, and obesity wasn't a widespread issue like it is today. Part of that reason is that they didn't eat all the processed foods and low-fat, low-calorie "diet" foods that we do today. So many people have messed up their metabolism by focusing on reducing calories that they ended up not getting the proper nutrition they needed to feed their body to stay slim and healthy. You can lose weight on 2,000 calories per day of clean, nutrient-rich foods and gain weight on 1,500 calories per day of junk food.

If you are used to counting calories and have had success with that method to help control your weight, then by all means continue counting calories. However, if you do not have success with counting calories, you'll want to focus on what you're eating, the type of foods you're eating, and how they affect your weight loss.

The Importance of Detoxifying to Lose Weight

Another reason traditional diets so often don't work is that they don't address the toxic waste in the body. Simply counting calories does not detoxify and cleanse the body. Weight loss won't be permanent if your body's systems are sluggish or impacted with waste matter or you suffer from toxic overload. In the DEM System, we ensure that you first rid your body of toxins, sludge, and excess waste to ensure that it can best utilize and metabolize the food you eat.

It is imperative that you detoxify the body to break the addiction to the foods that make you overweight and unhealthy in order to lose weight and keep it off. The method of dieting that involves resisting foods for a period of time and then returning to old eating habits will always cause the weight to return. Therefore, the goal is to break the addiction to foods that cause you to be overweight so you no longer desire or crave them anymore. Most traditional diets don't address how detoxifying the body aids in permanent weight loss.

Why Popular Diets Fail Us

There are many people who have tried popular diets but still struggle to lose the weight permanently. The primary reason is that most of the popular diets lack the nutritional support to allow your body to naturally regulate and lose weight. The diets often work in the short term, but they can also cause health problems, such as bloating, constipation, fatigue, or skin problems or make current health conditions worse due to the lack of balanced nutrition.

Additionally, these diets don't address the underlying hormonal imbalances and sluggish metabolism issues that cause weight gain. Let's look at some of the current and popular diets and why they don't work for permanent weight loss.

High-Protein/Low-Carb Diets. Some of the most popular diets of our generation involve reducing or eliminating the intake of carbohydrates. When you do this, you will lose weight, but eliminating an entire food group removes nutrients the body needs to function properly. On this type of diet, you can eat large amounts of protein and fat and still continue to lose weight.

The main problem with high-protein/low-carb diets is that they severely restrict an entire food group that has essential nutrients. Carbohydrates, such as grains, fruits, and vegetables, are what give us energy. When you stop eating carbohydrates, your body begins to break down fat very rapidly to receive a substitute for the carbohydrates it is no longer getting. This causes fat loss, initially. But your body will burn only a small amount of fat before it stops using fat as an energy source. It then begins to burn off water and then muscle tissue. In more serious cases, it will turn to connective tissue and then organ tissue. This process is called catabolism, and it can become extremely dangerous, even deadly. Eventually, melatonin and serotonin are not produced, which suppresses your ability to function normally and maintain energy. High-protein/low-carb diets can cause low energy, fatigue, sleeplessness, mental confusion, fainting, and vomiting. You will lose weight, but unfortunately, you will gain it back when you go off the diet.

Low-Fat Diets. Low-fat diets are among the most unsuccessful of all diets. Too many people focus on reducing and limiting all fat in their diet. We now know that healthy fats are a vital part of the body's survival and balance. The body's use of fat helps determine the satisfaction level a person receives from food. It helps to produce key hormones that assist with proper functioning of the brain.

When low-fat diets became popular, many companies began offering low-fat versions of their products. But if you read the labels, many of these low-fat foods actually contain more calories than the regular version. This is due to the sugar added to make up for the flavor that was lost when fat was eliminated from the product. If you eat these foods, you really aren't making much progress toward your weight-loss goals while on a low-fat diet. So many people end up eating low-fat foods and snacks thinking they were working towards losing weight, when in actuality they were eating more sugar and calories than they had in the past.

High-Carbohydrate Diets. A high-carb diet has a lot of potatoes, breads, pastas, grains, and rice—so-called "energy" foods. Although carbs are necessary for a well-balanced diet, too many carbs can have a negative effect on blood-sugar levels, which affects mood and brain functioning. Additionally, too many carbs can create a condition known as insulin resistance, which I'll discuss later. Insulin resistance is a common, but not widely known, reason so many people are getting fat at an alarming rate.

Additionally, carbs tend to have more calories than other foods. In the long term, a high-carb diet prevents the body from burning fat for fuel. So even though you may initially lose weight, you will quickly gain more weight, namely fat.

I have often said, it's not hard to lose weight rapidly, but the trick is to keep the weight off permanently. Permanent weight loss must come from burning fat and maintaining as much lean muscle mass as possible. You want to eliminate toxic overload in the body to shrink your fat cells. You want to also be sure that your hormones are properly balanced and that they are not hindering your weight-loss goals. Permanent weight loss (or fat loss) can be achieved with knowledge and effort as long as you remember that people don't fail at diets; diets fail people. Most diets simply don't help you achieve permanent weight loss.

CHAPTER TWO

Why Exercise Won't Make You Thin

I s exercising good for your health? Sure! Is it key to losing weight? Absolutely not! But so many people believe that it is. We've all heard the mantra "eat less and exercise more to lose weight." Close to 50 million Americans have gym memberships or belong to health clubs. We spend about $20 billion a year on gym memberships, yet obesity rates continue to drastically increase year after year.

There are many good reasons to exercise, such as improving cardiovascular health, but weight loss is not one of them. The truth of the matter is that although exercise is important for good health, the foods you eat are three times more important for controlling your weight than exercise. I remember reading a *Time* magazine cover story that quoted the prominent exercise researcher and professor, Eric Ravussin, who admitted to *Time* ("Why Exercise Won't Make You Thin," August 9, 2009) that "in general, for weight loss, exercise is pretty useless."

To lose one pound of fat by exercising, you must burn 3,500 calories. This would be equivalent to running thirty-five miles or walking on a treadmill for about seven and a half hours (at four miles per hour). As you can see, it would take a considerable amount of exercise to make a huge impact on your weight-loss goals.

I think it is important to note that exercise has many more benefits beyond weight loss. Most people who take up exercise become healthier by increasing their aerobic activity, which results in decreased blood pressure and overall better mood and mental health. I think because exercise is good for your overall health, many health practitioners downplay the fact that more and more research has shown that exercise has a negligible impact on weight loss. In other words, exercise may not be critical for weight loss, but in general, it is still great for our overall health.

It is true that exercise burns calories, and you must burn calories to lose weight, but exercise has another effect that counteracts the burning of calories: it stimulates hunger, which causes you to eat more, which in turn offsets any weight lost from exercising. Exercise doesn't necessarily make you lose weight; in fact, it could make you gain some. The one time in my life that I worked out with a trainer for a few months, I gained fifteen pounds. When I complained to my trainer, he said the extra weight was all muscle. But my feeling was *Who cares? I can't fit into my clothes.* And I hated my new body shape—not curvy and shapely, but big and bulky.

Even though I feel it is one of my personal flaws, I have to be honest with you: I don't work out. I haven't exercised in years. I tried to in the past but could never stick with it for more than four months, even when I had a trainer. I know that it's good for me and that we should all exercise, but unfortunately, I don't have the discipline to stick to an exercise regimen. However, I do have a strong desire to look and feel great. So I had to figure out how I could lose weight and keep it off, knowing that I didn't want to do fad diets and didn't want to be in the gym all the time. Happily, I found a system of healthy living that has yielded amazing results: permanent weight loss, a higher energy level, and overall great health! As a result, I have come to the conclusion that staying slim is all about eating right, while being fit is about exercising. So, as long as I focus on healthy eating, I will continue to stay slim. But if I want to reach a high level of fitness, I will need to incorporate more exercise into my life.

Focus on Physical Activity Throughout Each Day

The question we should be asking ourselves is how much physical activity we need to be healthy and fit. Physical activity is about movement—things that get you moving throughout the day and away from the computer, TV, bed, or couch. Exercise is a type of physical activity where you set aside a specified amount of time to get moving. You can be physically active throughout the course of the day without ever going to the gym.

People tend to greatly overestimate how many calories they burn while "exercising." The reality is that walking on a treadmill for about an hour burns only 350 to 400 calories, which can be nullified with one jelly donut or one or two glasses of wine. People typically burn 200 to 300 calories in a 30-minute aerobic-exercise session, but when they follow it up with a bottle of Gatorade, they replace all the calories they just burned. Another way to think of it is that you have to do a lot more exercise than the average person does in a typical hour-long session to burn off about 500 calories. To burn off just two donuts, about 500 calories, takes roughly two hours of cycling. To burn off two slices of pepperoni pizza, you'd have to do one and a half hours of swimming. So you have to do an awful lot more exercise than most people realize to make any real progress toward weight loss.

For some time, researchers have been finding that people who exercise don't necessarily lose weight. An increasing body of work reveals that exercise is rather ineffective when it comes to losing weight unless eating habits are also changed. Changing how and what you eat is the most effective route for losing weight. So, practically speaking, exercise is not the most effective method for slimming down unless you have the training regimen of an Olympian or professional athlete.

I definitely don't want to give people an excuse to not exercise; rather, I want them to accurately understand what exercise can and cannot do for their weight-loss goals. Those of you who do exercise should be proud of yourselves, and I encourage you to keep it up. When you get more physically active, you feel better about yourself and feel more inclined to watch the type of foods you put in your body.

In a very noteworthy experiment led by Dr. Timothy Church at the University of Louisiana, who published his results in the prestigious *Journal of the American Medical Association*, hundreds of overweight women were put on exercise regimens for a six-month period for the purpose of determining the health benefits of exercise. One group worked out for 70 minutes each week, another for 135 minutes, another for 190 minutes, and another kept to their normal daily routine with no additional exercise. The women in the study were all postmenopausal, sedentary, overweight, and had elevated blood pressure. To ensure there was 100 percent compliance with the exercise regimens, the women's exercising was supervised to accurately monitor results.

It was found that there was no significant difference in weight loss between those who had exercised, even with some groups exercising for several hours per week, and those who did not exercise. In fact, some of the women who exercised even gained weight. The possible reason for this was a problem identified as "compensation." Those who did exercise cancelled out the calories they had just burned by eating more, typically as a self-reward (rewarding yourself with food) for working out or to satisfy their stimulated appetites from the actual workout. It would be as if I would eat a donut or pastry to celebrate all the hard effort that I just put in during my workout, but in reality, I simply erased all the calories that were burned. So, if you have committed to exercising, and that is indeed a good thing, be sure not to get in the habit of rewarding yourself with food.

One positive finding in the study was that every exercise group reported an improvement in quality of life, including the group that exercised for ten minutes a day. That means that as little as ten minutes of exercise a day has benefits. This is very good news for those who can find only ten to fifteen minutes a day for exercise but are not able to find one hour, three times a week.

Barry Braun, associate professor of kinesiology at the

University of Massachusetts, found that the evidence emerging from his research team shows that moderate exercise, such as "low-intensity ambulation" (i.e., walking), may help to burn calories "without triggering a caloric compensation effect," meaning you won't immediately feel the need for a snack after your workout as a result of increased appetite hormones in your blood. This means that an intense workout in the gym might actually be less effective than gentle exercises, such as walking, in terms of weight loss because you don't get the stimulated appetite that comes with intense workouts.

If you look at numerous studies over the years, it clearly shows exercise alone won't make you thin; rather, being physically active is a key factor in weight loss. In the DEM System, we focus on ways to get physically active throughout the day as opposed to just exercising a few times a week. Even if you just do light exercise—like taking a brisk walk to and from lunch or walking up the stairs instead of taking the elevator—you will get many of the good benefits of exercise. This is because light exercise can increase your heart rate and improve your cardiovascular health.

Another consideration is that once you become overweight, it is much harder to exercise or go to the gym to work out. However, you are more likely to be able to simply "get moving" throughout the day. Once you begin to lose weight and become healthier, it will be easier to incorporate more intense physical activity (i.e., exercise) into your daily regimen.

I strongly believe that nutritional education must come first. People don't lack willpower; they lack nutritional education. Eating habits must change first with a focus on nutrient-rich foods that do not cause the body to gain and store fat. I believe that changing how and what you eat will help you lose weight. Being physically active helps you keep the weight off permanently, so you'll find two key steps of the DEM System are to EAT (healthy, nutrient-rich foods) and to MOVE (get physically active throughout the day). Since we know being physically active is good for your overall health, it makes sense to focus on that as well as changing your eating habits.

CHAPTER THREE

Why a Sugar Addiction Is Worse Than a Drug Addiction

M
any people are addicted to sugar and don't even know it. I believe this addiction is the main reason people get fat. They don't think they eat a lot of sugar because they don't eat a lot of candy, cakes, and pies, but the problem is that sugar is hidden in many foods, including breads, muffins, and even dried fruit. I believe sugar is toxic. It has no nutritional value, it's highly addictive, and it makes you sick and fat.

Certain types of foods, such as processed foods and simple carbohydrates (candy, sugar, sweets), are high in sugar, toxic to our digestive system, and cause us to gain weight and make poor food choices in the long run. Processed foods and simple carbohydrates (sugar) are low in nutrients and high in calories. Many of us have heard that excess sugar consumption can lead to food cravings, binge eating, and, worst of all, sugar addiction. Sugar stimulates the dopamine and opioid receptors of the brain, which are the same receptors stimulated by other addictive substances, such as cocaine and morphine. Just like those drugs, sugar can become addictive. If you try to cut back or break your addiction to sugar, you will experience withdrawal symptoms, the same as a drug addict does. Over time, having an excess of refined sugar in the diet leads to not only weight gain but also other serious diseases, like heart disease, stroke, or type-2 diabetes.

Dr. Judith J. Wurtman, a nutritionist at MIT, has shown that eating refined carbohydrates like cookies, cakes, candy, pasta, or white bread raises serotonin and endorphins in the brain, creating a happy, feel-good, peaceful state. This is why we crave these carbs when we're anxious or stressed. However, you only "feel good" in the short term and then you crave more in order to remain in that happy state. You begin self-medicating with food— eating sweets to make yourself feel balanced and calm. No matter if you crave sweets or breads or pasta, it all has the same effect because it all converts quickly to sugar in your body and causes you to crave more of the same.

How Sugar Makes You Fat

When you eat sugar, it gets stored in the liver in the form of glycogen. When the liver is overloaded with sugar, it begins to expand, and when it is maxed out, the glycogen is expelled in the form of fatty acids. This excess fat—called fatty acid—is deposited into areas such as the belly, butt, thighs, and hips. Where it gets most dangerous is when the remaining fatty acids end up in our major organs, including the heart and kidneys.

Sugary foods (candy, cakes, pies, muffins, and sodas) and other refined, starchy carbohydrates cause a rapid rise in insulin levels, which results in excess fat in the body. When food is eaten, it is broken down to glucose so it can be used to fuel the body. Insulin is the hormone that sends glucose out of the blood into the tissue cells for use as energy. When excess glucose remains in the blood, insulin levels stay high. Chronically elevated insulin can cause both fat storage and more inflammation in the body. When insulin levels are high, this is a signal to the body to store extra calories as fat and to refrain from burning fat. High insulin levels mean you'll have more body fat, while low insulin levels mean you'll have less body fat.

Research has also shown that a high-sugar diet causes cancer cells to multiply rapidly. An important study published in the medical journal *Cancer Research* was conducted by a team out of the University of California, Los Angeles. The researchers found that while sugar of any kind offered sustenance to cancer cells, fructose sugar played a key role in the proliferation of cancer cells. That means that cancer spreads more quickly on a high-fructose sugar diet.

The food industry has been extremely successful at designing foods to capture the hearts and minds of those who enjoy food. Food manufacturers and restaurant owners may not fully understand the science behind why sugar, salt, and fat sell so well, but they know that they do. Thus, they make foods that are laden with sugar, salt, and fat. When food appeals to our taste buds, we say that it is palatable. But scientists know that food that is palatable stimulates our appetite and cravings and causes us to eat more of it. In fact, we become motivated to pursue that taste over and over again. Eating foods high in sugar and salt makes us want to eat more foods that are high in sugar and salt. Eating foods that taste good causes us to eat more food that tastes good.

The average American's sugar load is about 100 pounds

per year. We have become physically addicted to simple carbohydrates (candy, sugar, sweets). In a 2007 study conducted in France, cocaine-addicted rats were offered super-sweetened water using a combination of sugar and artificial sweeteners. In just three days, the cocaine-addicted rats switched their allegiance from cocaine to the super-sweetened sugar water. The conclusion was that sugar activates dopamine receptors just as cocaine does. But unlike cocaine, sugar has no adverse effects on the nervous system. When the rats got a hit of sugar, they gained the highs of cocaine without the downside of increased nervousness. Since cocaine is known to be one of the most addictive substances on earth, we can see how humans can so easily get addicted to sugar. Sugar gives them the same effect of the hit on their dopamine receptors as cocaine does. Humans can easily become addicted to sugar and go through withdrawal if they can't get sugar quickly.

Are You Addicted to Sugar?

If you answer yes to more than ten of these questions, then chances are that you are a *sugar addict*.

- ☐ Do you put sugar in coffee or tea?
- ☐ Do you drink sodas at least once a day?
- ☐ Do you drink sweetened fruit punches, sports drinks, or juices?
- ☐ Do you use syrups, jams, or jellies several times a week?
- ☐ Did you eat a lot of candy growing up as a kid?
- ☐ Do you crave sweets, pasta, or breads or are they your favorite foods?

- [ ] Do you eat bread, bagels, croissants, muffins, or donuts for breakfast?
- [ ] Do you feel chronically tired or fatigued most days?
- [ ] Do you often eat a dessert after dinner?
- [ ] Do you crave sweets in the afternoon or late at night?
- [ ] Do you buy candy at the movie theater?
- [ ] Do you have headaches often?
- [ ] Do you drink fruity or sweetened alcoholic drinks?
- [ ] Do you keep candy or snacks in your home at all times?
- [ ] Do you eat sweets first at a happy hour or party?

There are so many good reasons to break your sugar addiction, but at the top of the list is that sugar makes you fat and it makes you sick.

How to Break the Sugar Addiction

Are you having a panic attack right now just thinking about giving up sugar? You have to look at kicking the sugar habit as though you are ending an addiction. The key is to understand where your sugar is coming from and then find alternatives to eating so much sugar in your foods.

Start by making yourself aware of everything that has sugar in it. First, you must know how to find sugar in your foods, as it is cleverly hidden in the labeling. Virtually everything we eat, especially packaged and processed foods—including diet and low-fat foods—has sugar in it.

You will want to read labels to determine the total amount of sugar in the products you buy and to check the list of ingredients for the names of things that are really just sugar in disguise. Refined white sugar, or table sugar, which is sucrose, is the form of sugar that is most familiar to people. However, the other sugars that are commonly found in food are listed on labels as high-fructose corn syrup, glucose, fructose (fruit sugar), dextrose (corn sugar), maltose (malt sugar), lactose (milk sugar), corn sweetener, raw sugar, brown sugar, powdered sugar, molasses, and maple sugar.

Begin by looking at your drinks and the packaged goods in your refrigerator and pantry. Get rid of those foods that have a high sugar content (5 grams of sugar or more per serving).

Sugar is measured in grams, and 4 grams of sugar equals one teaspoon. So if your soda has 40 grams of sugar, that's about ten teaspoons of sugar in just one soda. You can see how so many people end up eating so much sugar every day. I used to think I was eating a healthy breakfast by eating oatmeal. However, it wasn't regular oatmeal but the sweetened, flavored instant oatmeal, like apple-cinnamon oatmeal, and it had about 20 grams of sugar per serving, which is way too much.

Remember, as a guideline, the best way to minimize the amount of sugar in your diet is to choose foods that have 5 grams or less per serving. When the drink or food item has 5 grams or less of sugar per serving size, the body doesn't overreact to the sugar. This means your pancreas will not have to release too much insulin, which can cause fat storage in the body. (I'll explain this concept in a later chapter.)

To sweeten foods, it is always better to use stevia or some equivalent herbal sweetener rather than sugar. Stevia is a natural sweetener made from a plant native to South America and Central America. Other countries have been using stevia as a sugar substitute for several decades since it is virtually calorie-free and does not affect blood glucose, which makes it a great natural alternative to sugar and artificial sweeteners.

When you crave sweets, try fruit as a better alternative. In fact, it is your best defense against insulin spikes and cravings. Facing these cravings is the beginning of detoxifying and rebalancing your body. The cravings will actually disappear after three to four days. And once you fight these cravings, your cravings won't be as strong as long as you continue to keep high-sugar foods out of your diet.

Sugar will cause you to get fat, feel irritable, moody, and tired, and can cause all kinds of health problems, so commit to breaking your sugar addiction today!

CHAPTER FOUR

How Toxins Make You Fat, Sick, and Tired

was coaching a client a few weeks ago, and she asked me a very poignant question: "JJ, why am I always sick, and what's making me fat?" I said, "That is not the question of the day, but the question of the century." Toxins make us fat and sick! And they are the missing piece to the puzzle as to why we can't lose weight and why we feel unhealthy and tired!

What Are Toxins?

A toxin is any substance that irritates or creates harmful effects in the body or mind. Toxins are everywhere, and we are unknowingly filling our bodies with them every day. There are two types of toxins: environmental toxins and internal toxins.

- Environmental toxins are found outside the body/mind and include pollutants, smog, medications, hormones/birth control pills, household cleaners, food additives, and pesticides.

- Internal toxins are found inside the body/mind and include bacterial/yeast/fungal overgrowth, parasite infections, chronic worry or fear, food allergies, and dental or medical implants, such as implants from cosmetic surgeries, joint replacements, or mercury dental fillings.

We live in a sea of toxins. You cannot avoid them, but you can help your body get rid of some of them. Every person on the planet has residues of toxic chemicals or metals in their tissues. Some 80,000 new chemicals have been introduced since the turn of the twentieth century, and most have never been tested for safety or for how they interact in the human body. Our air is toxic; our water is polluted; our food is depleted of nutrients and packed with poisonous chemicals and hormones. Not only that, but our minds and hearts often get polluted also.

Toxins create a heavy burden in the body, which causes many of the body's systems to malfunction. The buildup of toxins overwhelms the body's vital organs and other systems, creating an array of health issues, including fatigue, memory loss, premature aging, skin eruptions/acne, depression, arthritis, hormone imbalances, chronic fatigue, anxiety, emotional disorders, muscle and joint pain, cancers, heart disease, and much, much more.

There's no delicate way of putting this, but to some extent, we're all toxic, which is one of the biggest reasons so many people are overweight. Just because you are overweight does not guarantee that you have a toxic overload, and just because you are thin does not mean that you do not have a toxic overload. We have to evaluate our toxic overload individually, regardless of whether we are slim or fat. However, it is rare that an overweight person who rids the body of excess toxins does not lose weight. Please know that getting rid of the fat by exercising or dieting doesn't necessarily get rid of the toxins. Toxins just get reabsorbed by your body, creating new fat cells, which makes losing weight without getting rid of the toxins a hinder to permanent weight loss.

Some research data implies that the obesity epidemic in the United States is due to toxic overload. An article in the April 2002 issue of *The Journal of Alternative and Complementary Medicine* concluded the following: "The commonly held causes of obesity such as overeating and inactivity do not explain the current obesity epidemic. Because the obesity epidemic occurred rather quickly, it has been suggested that environmental causes instead of genetic factors may be largely responsible." In other words, they are suggesting that the environmental chemicals (i.e., toxins) that have increased in number over the last one hundred years may help explain the widespread obesity epidemic.

Having monitored human exposure to toxic environmental chemicals since 1972, the Environmental Protection Agency (EPA) began the National Human Adipose Tissue Survey to evaluate the levels of various toxins in fat tissue. The study found that five of what are known to be the most toxic chemicals (OCDD or octachlorodibenzo-p-dioxin, styrene, dichlorobenzene, xylene, and ethylphenol) were found in 100 percent of all tissue samples. These toxic chemicals from industrial pollution damage the liver, heart, lungs, and nervous system. Additionally, nine more chemicals were found in 91 to 98 percent of samples, including benzene, toluene, ethylbenzene, and DDE. These toxins found in the fat tissues not only contribute to our weight issues but are also damaging our health.

The good news is that one way to get rid of excess toxins in the body is by changing the thing that caused it in the first place, which is diet. In the DEM System, we provide foods that help you rid the body of toxins, resulting in improved energy, health, and vitality.

Toxic Overload in Your Body

Toxic overload refers to the level of toxins found in tissues of the human body by analysis of the blood and urine. Toxins are stored in almost every tissue in the body, including fat, skeletal muscle, bones, tendons, joints/ligaments, and visceral organs.

When the body is properly nourished and detoxified, its organs operate at peak performance. However, whenever our elimination channels become clogged due to toxic overload and poor diet, we should follow a comprehensive detoxification program to improve its functioning. Detoxification may still be unfamiliar to many but is really quite natural and beneficial. Just as we regularly clean our homes, our cars, and the outside of our bodies, we should cleanse our inner body.

First, to get a sense of what the toxic load is in your body, take the "How Toxic Are You?" Quiz.

How Toxic Are You? Quiz

If you are dealing with fatigue, weight gain, chronic disease, inability to focus, or accelerated aging, you will want to take this quiz to determine if toxic overload in your body is the underlying cause. Take this quiz and score your results to gain a sense of how much toxic burden you're carrying in your body.

Read each question and give yourself one point for every *yes* answer.

- ☐ Do you crave sweets, bread, pasta, white rice, and/or potatoes?
- ☐ Do you eat processed foods (TV dinners, lunch-meat) or fast foods at least three times a week?
- ☐ Do you drink caffeinated beverages like coffee and tea more than twice daily?
- ☐ Do you drink diets sodas or use artificial sweeteners at least once a day?
- ☐ Do you sleep less than eight hours per day?
- ☐ Do you drink less than 64 ounces of good, clean water daily?
- ☐ Are you very sensitive to smoke, chemicals, or fumes in the environment?
- ☐ Have you or are you taking antibiotics, antidepressants, or other medications?
- ☐ Do you or have you taken birth control pills or other estrogens, such as hormone replacement therapy?
- ☐ Do you have frequent yeast infections?
- ☐ Do you have "silver" dental fillings?
- ☐ Do you use commercial household cleaners, cosmetics, or deodorants?
- ☐ Do you eat non-organic vegetables, fruits, or meat?
- ☐ Have you ever smoked or been exposed to secondhand smoke?

☐ Are you overweight or do you have cellulite fat deposits?

☐ Does your occupation expose you to environmental toxins?

☐ Do you live in a major metropolitan city or near a big airport?

☐ Do you feel tired, fatigued, or sluggish throughout the day?

☐ Do you have difficulty concentrating or focusing?

☐ Do you suffer bloating, indigestion, or frequent gas after eating?

☐ Do you get more than two colds or the flu per year?

☐ Do you have reoccurring congestion, sinus issues, or postnasal drip?

☐ Do you sometimes notice bad breath, a coated tongue, or strong-smelling urine?

☐ Do you have puffy eyes or dark circles under your eyes?

☐ Are you often sad or depressed?

☐ Do you often feel anxious, antsy, or stressed?

☐ Do you have acne, breakouts, rashes, or hives?

☐ Do you have less than one bowel movement per day and/or get constipated occasionally?

☐ Do you have insomnia or trouble getting restful sleep?

☐ Do you get blurred vision or itchy, burning eyes?

The higher your score, the greater the potential toxic burden you may be carrying and the more you may benefit from a detoxification and cleansing program. If you scored twenty or higher, you will *significantly* benefit from detoxifying your body, which could lead to weight loss and improved health and vitality. If you scored between five and nineteen, you may benefit from a detoxification program for improved health and vitality. If you scored below five, you might actually be free of toxic overload in the body and living a very healthy, toxin-free life. Good for you!

Signs of toxic overload in the body include the following:

- Bloating and gas
- Constipation
- Indigestion
- Low energy /fatigue
- Brain fog/depression
- Weight gain
- Chronic pain
- Infections
- Allergies
- Headaches

Toxic overload can also be identified through different tests that help determine your individual body burden. There are facilities that offer specialty testing that measure toxicity levels. Look for those that are CLIA-certified by the Centers of Medicaid and Medicare Services. Other services offered to the general public can be found through companies such as LabSafe.com and

LabTestingDirect.com. Through these companies, you can take a variety of laboratory tests, including over forty different tests for toxins. The cost to determine the toxic overload in your body ranges from $100 to $400.

One of the most commonly held myths today is that the body can detoxify itself and does not need any help. You may have heard that the body can eliminate toxins on its own. Our body does naturally try to eliminate toxins, but overexposure to any of them will slow down the body's detoxification systems. The reality is that you can assist the body in detoxifying and eliminating toxins that cause weight gain and harm your health. You can and should detoxify and cleanse the body if you want to live better and live longer. Yes, toxins are real, they do exist, and the good news is that there are many ways to eliminate them from the body. In this book, I will provide the most practical and effective techniques to detoxify and cleanse the body.

Many people struggle on a diet because of their strong cravings. Cravings are not only a matter of willpower. They can actually be eliminated by properly detoxing and cleansing the body to eliminate waste and toxins. As I gained weight in my thirties, I learned that although my metabolism was beginning to slow due to aging, that wasn't the real reason why I couldn't lose weight. I learned that my excess weight was not all fat; some of it was waste in my body—excess toxic waste caused by years of poor eating, leading to fluid retention and intestinal waste matter in my colon.

Many in the medical industry will tell you that you do not need to help your body cleanse and detoxify. Yet, there is more and more scientific research that shows industrial and environmental toxins to be a factor in many diseases, such as Parkinson's. Most of the advice that comes from the medical community around weight loss focuses on eating less and exercising more. But I never trust my health and wellness solely to the medical community and really feel that I don't need a license in order to understand my body and health. I have the ultimate respect for doctors, but in my opinion, they are trained to treat symptoms and may not be as experienced in understanding the role toxic overload plays on our health issues and ailments. This is true, particularly if a doctor received his medical degree decades ago.

However, as with any change to your diet or lifestyle, you should consult with your physician as you begin your journey toward healthy eating and living. In fact, you may even enlighten him and provide valuable information that he can utilize in his practice to help other patients. We are all here to help one another toward great health. One of my favorite quotes is the following: "Health is a state of complete physical, mental, and social well-being and not merely the absence of disease or infirmity" (World Health Organization, 1948).

How Our Standard American Diet (SAD) Contributes to Toxic Overload in the Body

An important link between weight gain and toxic overload in the body is the quality of the food we eat. Food is our energy source, and the more nutritional the food, the better the body will function. If we choose foods that are nutrient-rich, organic, and free of toxins, the body will receive and absorb the highest nutrient intake, allowing us to feel satisfied and full without empty calories, which cause us to eat more and more. Yet we are eating less and less of these healthy, nutrient-rich foods today.

The Standard American Diet (SAD) consists of highly processed and refined foods, including frozen foods, fast foods, and prepared foods that are canned, boxed, and processed to create "instant" varieties that are the least healthy for you. Restaurants, especially fast-food chains, and supermarkets are filled with foods high in fat, sugar, cholesterol, sodium, artificial flavors, pesticides, hormones, and preservatives, all of which contribute to the toxic over-load in the body.

Let's take a closer look at the Standard American Diet that so many of us eat. It typically includes lots of highly refined wheat products, such as white bread, crackers, bagels, pasta, and cereals, as well as other processed foods, such as potato chips and corn chips. Don't forget the fatty meats like steaks, burgers, hot dogs, ribs, bacon, and pork chops. Now, top it all off with a large amount of saturated fat, hydrogenated oil, and processed vegetable oils, such as salad dressing, most cooking oils, and mayonnaise. It's no wonder we have an epidemic of heart disease, cancer, diabetes, and arthritis as well as many other degenerative diseases. Now, for dessert, we eat baked goods, such as cakes, pies, cupcakes, cookies, fudge, and brownies—and don't forget the donuts and candy bars. In many ways, former generations were some of the healthiest people on the planet because many of these foods did not exist. But today, our lifestyle has become much too stressed and fast-paced to take time to eat healthy foods. However, we are supposed to eat in order to "feed" our body the nutrients it needs to maintain vitality and health.

It's not just how much you're eating that's causing you to gain weight, it is also what you're eating and what you're body is being exposed to that causes a toxic overload in your body. Even though we are not technically starving like some people in other areas of the world, we are definitely malnourished. We eat a lot, but our nutritional deficiencies manifest themselves as "belly fat," "thunder thighs," "underarm bat wings," "beer bellies," and "cottage cheese behind." Do any of these sound familiar?

How Toxins Cause Excess Fat in the Body

There are many factors that contribute to weight gain, and one factor that is most overlooked by traditional diets is toxic overload. Simply put, people often have difficulty losing weight because their bodies are full of poisons. The more toxins you take in or are exposed to every day, the more toxins you store in fat cells in the body. Toxins stored in fat cells are difficult to get rid of through dieting alone. You must first detoxify the body. When the body is overloaded with toxins, the body transfers its energy away from burning calories and uses that energy to work harder to detoxify the body. In other words, the body does not have the energy to burn calories. However, when the body is efficiently detoxifying and getting rid of toxins, the energy can be used to burn fat. Thus, the DEM System starts with detoxification as the first step in helping you shed pounds.

I believe the most effective weight-loss programs should focus on both fat loss and detoxification. Detoxification, which is the process of removing toxins from the body, is critical to losing fat because many of the toxins the body holds onto are stored in fat cells. When you begin to lose weight (fat), toxins stored in fat cells are released into the bloodstream and need to be eliminated from the body so they don't cause illness. Therefore, weight loss that includes detoxification results in not only fat loss but also overall improved health and wellness.

Your body stores the majority of toxins in fat cells, and it's actually safer for toxins to be in your fat cells than in your bloodstream. The downside to this is that the more body fat you have, the more toxins you are also storing. And because your body knows that releasing toxins into your bloodstream is less desirable than having them stored safely in your fat cells, it holds on to the fat cells for dear life and doesn't want to let them go, making it difficult for you to lose fat. Thus, fat cells don't break down very easily and they literally weigh down the body and make it bigger.

So, the first step in losing weight is detoxification. Without detoxification, millions of people worldwide lose the fight to lose weight permanently. The more toxins the body is storing, the more fat it is likely to accumulate and retain. It is not by accident that American obesity levels are rising right alongside the increase in environmental toxins.

How Toxins Hinder Weight Loss

A study published in *Obesity Reviews* concluded that during weight loss, certain toxins (e.g., pesticides) are released from fat tissue where they are typically stored. These toxins can pollute your body, slow metabolism, and make additional weight loss more challenging. Additional studies suggest toxins released during weight loss interfere with thyroid and mitochondrial function, which disrupts your metabolic rate and reduces your body's ability to burn fat and calories. A study by Catherine Pelletier, a researcher at Laval University, supports how environmental toxins can also negatively affect your thyroid, which is critical for proper metabolism regulation. So it becomes imperative to take steps to detoxify the body if you plan to lose weight and excess body fat. This will allow for safer toxin elimination and avoid the slowing of your metabolism.

Toxins can interfere with your ability to lose weight by:

- *Slowing down your metabolism.* As toxins are being released from fat cells, they may cause the thyroid to slow down, negatively impacting metabolism. When the thyroid slows down, so does metabolism, which leads to weight gain and low energy.

- *Decreasing your ability to burn fat.* Toxins hinder the body's ability to burn fat by up to 20 percent. Toxins released during weight loss interfere with mitochondrial function, which reduces your body's ability to burn fat.

- *Slowing down the time it takes for you to feel full.* There are hormones that send signals that tell the brain we are full so that we stop eating. Toxic overload causes hormonal imbalances that stop these signals from working properly.

- *Interfering with our appetite systems.* Besides directly lowering thyroid hormone levels, metabolic rate, and fat burning, toxins can damage the mechanisms that control appetite. Toxins can interfere with all the delicate appetite-control systems that are regulated by hormones and neurotransmitters from the fat cells, the gut, and brain.

43

Weight loss can be a challenge on its own, but when we add the fact that toxins residing in fat cells also play a factor, it is that much harder. If you had been making good progress losing weight and all of the sudden reached a plateau and can't lose those last twenty pounds, you may want to determine if toxic overload in your body is hindering your weight-loss progress.

PART 2

The Five Keys to Permanent Weight Loss

The Five Keys to Permanent Weight Loss

T here are five commandments to follow to achieve permanent weight loss, and all of them are addressed in the DEM System to ensure that you lose weight and keep it off. The five commandments are as follows:

1. Detoxify your body, primarily the liver, which must be able to properly metabolize sugars and fats so you can eliminate stubborn fat in the body.

2. Correct your hormonal imbalances so that your brain and gut communicate with one another to drive your eating behavior and control your appetite.

3. Learn how to accelerate your metabolism (metabolic engine) to turn your body into a fat-burning machine.

4. Eat foods that make you thin.

5. Avoid foods that make you fat.

Understanding the reasons for these five commandments will help you succeed not only in maintaining your ideal weight but also in managing your long-term health and even reversing chronic ailments and diseases. The consequence of these changes will result in effortless weight loss and a new feeling of life and renewed energy. You will enjoy delicious, healthy, nutritionist-designed food choices that have many fat-burning and healing properties.

Following these commandments is critical to long-term, sustainable weight loss that doesn't depend on eating less but rather on eating more nutrient-rich foods that help your body stay slim and healthy. While weight-loss experts have emphasized one or two of these elements, no one has integrated these five critical success factors into a complete program until now. Following the DEM System will ensure you permanent weight loss and good health for the rest of your life.

CHAPTER FIVE

Get Rid of Toxic Overload in the Body

As discussed in the previous chapter, the first key to weight loss involves getting rid of toxins in the body. If you try to lose weight without getting rid of the toxins, then you're guaranteed to gain the weight right back—even if you exercise to burn fat. To lose weight permanently, you must detoxify and cleanse the body to get rid of toxins we encounter every day so they don't reenter the body and create more and more fat cells.

What Does It Mean to Detoxify the Body?

Detoxification is a total-body cleansing process for all of the body's detoxification organs and systems. Detoxification is the process of cleansing and reducing the toxic overload that currently resides in your body. Because there are so many toxins in your cells, tissues, and organs, you detoxify to bring them out of hiding so they can be eliminated from the body.

Many people falsely think of the word "cleanse" as a one-time fast or colon cleanse you do for a few days every few years. This is detoxification in a very narrow sense. Although the colon is one of the many detoxification channels for elimination, total body cleansing goes far beyond colon cleansing.

It involves cleansing all of the detox organs, including the liver, kidneys, skin, etc. Just as you wouldn't wait a year to clean your house, you shouldn't wait a year to "cleanse" your inner body. Regular cleansing ensures that you are constantly eliminating toxins and getting rid of waste and sludge. If you wait too long to cleanse the body, toxins get deeper into the body, making you look and feel tired and old, eventually leading to disease and weight gain. The goal is not to be camped out near a toilet all day, but rather to incorporate detoxification methods that are gradual but steady to avoid disruptive side effects. Thus, we have to think of cleansing as a regular, ongoing activity we do to reach our highest potential for optimum health and wellness.

Detoxing differs from dieting in that its primary goal is to cleanse the entire body. However, one of the natural outcomes of detoxing is that excess weight melts away. The idea is to simply help the body in its natural process of self-cleansing.

We are continually eliminating excess toxins through our digestive, urinary, skin, circulatory, respiratory, and lymphatic systems. Helping the body cleanse is not unnatural. Some call the act of toxins being released from the tissues and cells "detoxification" while flushing the waste out or eliminating toxins from the body is "cleansing." For our purposes, we will refer to the entire process as detoxification or cleansing. In this book, the words detoxification, detox, and cleansing may be used interchangeably.

The benefits of detoxifying the body include:

- Weight loss and the realization that you can enjoy a lighter style of eating.

- Improved digestion; better elimination; less constipation, gas, bloating, and indigestion.

- Fewer allergic or reactive responses to foods.

- Less mucus and congestion and the clearing up of sniffles and coughs.

- More energy, better nutrient absorption, and overall improved health.

- Sense of satisfaction, greater vitality, and a desire to choose better foods and develop better eating habits, permanently.

How Does the Body Detoxify Itself?

Keep in mind that detoxification is a continuous process that happens in the body every day all day. We're constantly eliminating toxins through our digestive, urinary, skin, circulatory, respiratory, and lymphatic systems, and they all work well. However, as we get older, they don't function at peak performance due to toxic overload in the body.

The body has seven channels of elimination: the blood, the lymphatic system, and five organs—the colon, kidneys, lungs, skin, and liver. All have a unique role to play in getting rid of toxins and wastes, and all must be functioning optimally for effective total-body cleansing. However, the toxic overload in the body means these organs and systems may require assistance to meet the extra demand we put on them.

Let's take a look at the major detoxification organs and systems in the body.

- *Colon.* The colon is about six feet long and is the part of the body's digestive system that moves waste material from the small intestine to the rectum. The small intestine sucks all the nutrients out of what you eat and then passes the leftover waste to the large intestine, which is part of the colon. As the colon transports the waste material toward the rectum, it absorbs water from the waste. It may also absorb harmful materials. The longer it takes for waste to pass through the colon, the greater the chance of absorbing such harmful materials back into the body. This is why it is important to have regular, daily bowel movements to keep waste moving out of the body.

- *Kidneys.* The kidneys, which are located on either side of the lower back, are responsible for filtering the blood in the body and removing materials that the body does not require. These wastes and extra water become urine, which flows to the bladder for release.

- *Lungs.* Each day, you take about 23,000 breaths, which bring almost 10,000 quarts of air into your lungs. The air that you breathe in contains several gases, including oxygen, which your cells need to function. With each breath, your lungs add fresh oxygen to your blood, which then carries it to your cells.

- *Skin.* The skin, as the largest organ of the body, is one of our most efficient detoxification organs. Although the liver and kidneys are the primary sources of detoxification, the skin definitely plays an important role as well. When the body is detoxing properly, the skin excretes water and toxins, salt, and other chemicals from our body via sweat. The glands that are connected to millions of tiny hair follicles found in the pores of our skin produce sweat, allowing toxins to be released. We can monitor the state of our overall health by the skin. When our skin has a healthy glow and it's soft to the touch, it indicates that our body is detoxifying properly. In contrast, when our skin has dry patches, acne, hives, and rashes, it indicates that our internal organs are becoming overwhelmed with toxins.

- *Liver.* The liver, which is the largest of the internal organs, has the most important and comprehensive jobs of all the organs. It has a filtering capacity of one quart of blood every minute, and it has unique metabolic functions. As blood flows through the liver, the detoxification process begins. The liver excretes its toxins in the bile. The bile that is produced by the liver is actually stored in the gallbladder. It then empties the toxins into the small intestine, and they are eventually eliminated through the colon. However, if you are constipated, these toxins and bile may remain in the intestines too long. This causes toxic poisons that should be eliminated from the body to actually be reabsorbed into the body. These toxins can be stored for months or even years, but they can also be released when you perspire, like with exercise or in a sauna, which are excellent ways to excrete toxins through the skin. There will be much more discussion on the liver later in this chapter.

- *Lymphatic System.* The lymphatic system is a secondary circulatory system that supports detoxification and the immune system. The lymphatic system transports toxins and excess fluid, and our sweat glands release toxins through the skin. As tissues become filled with toxins from normal bodily functions, our bodies remove them by carrying them through the bloodstream to be processed by the liver. This occurs through the lymphatic system, which also transports fats and fatty acids as well as immune cells. In a healthy body, the lymphatic system works smoothly and efficiently, but once the body is overloaded with toxins, the lymphatic system can get backed up. Signs that the lymphatic system is working improperly are swelling in the hands, feet, and legs, and cellulite— yes, cellulite, ladies. In Chapter 14, we discuss some natural ways to get rid of cellulite.

The Primary Organ That Makes You Fat or Skinny

The one secret to losing weight and keeping it off is to keep the liver healthy and operating at peak performance. The liver (also known as the fat-burning organ) is the number-one secret weapon to weight loss. The liver is responsible for breaking down, eliminating, and neutralizing toxins in the body and breaking down fats in the body.

The liver, which is about the size of a football and weighs in at about three to five pounds, is the largest single organ in the body. Think of the liver as a washing machine for blood. The liver supports the digestive system, controls blood sugar levels, and regulates fat storage. If poisons or excess fats clog your liver, it can't perform its fat-burning function. When your liver cannot metabolize well, you have no energy, you won't absorb nutrients essential for your body to live, and your body can't fight disease.

The liver is responsible for a large variety of health-promoting functions that restore good health and help to maintain weight loss. The liver has all of the following functions:

- It filters your blood to remove toxins such as viruses, bacteria, yeast, and other poisonous foreign substances. When the liver is performing optimally, it can clear 99 percent of toxins from the blood before that blood is distributed to the rest of the body.

- It metabolizes fats by producing bile, a substance that breaks down fats so they can be digested. Daily, your liver produces about a quart of bile, which helps to digest dietary fats by breaking them down so they can be used as fuel.

- It metabolizes carbohydrates and helps the body maintain healthy levels of blood sugar.

- It breaks down proteins into their amino acid parts, creating vital blood proteins.

- It acts as a large storage unit, housing an abundance of substances, including glycogen for stored energy, iron, blood, and vitamins A, D, and B12.

- It keeps your metabolic engines running and your body free of toxins, removing drugs, chemicals, and hormones from the blood—deactivating and eliminating them.

In today's environment, we take in more and more toxins every day: pollutants, birth control pills, prescription medications, household cleaners, food additives, and pesticides. As we age, toxins build up in our system and create a toxic overload in the body. When the liver is overloaded with toxins, it has a difficult time eliminating them, so it begins to store them in fat cells. The more toxins we take in over time, the more fat cells are created in the body.

When your liver functions efficiently, it is much easier for you to lose weight. The liver has to perform well enough to eliminate the toxins that are causing fat cells in the body. If you have body fat accumulation, especially around the waist and midsection (i.e., belly fat), it suggests that your liver may not be functioning properly or as efficiently as it could. To lose this excess weight, you have to detoxify and cleanse the liver, which leads to not only a slimmer waistline but also a thinner body.

The most common liver disease in America is a condition known as fatty liver disease, in which the liver stops processing fat and begins storing it right around the waistline. Fatty liver disease affects 20 percent of the population. The major cause of fatty liver disease is overconsumption of sugar, high-fructose corn syrup, and refined carbohydrates (like white flour, white rice, and white sugar). Excess sugar also damages the mitochondria. Mitochondria are the tiny power producers within each cell that convert sugar into energy. As we age, mitochondria become less numerous and less efficient. Each cell has over 1,000 mitochondria when you are young, but less than half that number by the time you are fifty. This means your body produces less energy, resulting in a slower metabolism. One of the principle reasons we gain weight as we age is that our bodies produce less energy, yet we continue to have the same energy intake from food. A fatty liver is also an inflamed liver, producing more inflammatory molecules throughout the body, which leads to more mitochondrial damage. Preventing mitochondrial damage is critical to sustaining weight loss. When the mitochondria are damaged, we can't effectively burn fat or calories, resulting in a slower metabolism and more weight gain.

I know, you might be thinking *I believe my liver is working just fine.* But how do you know? Some of the symptoms of toxic overload in the body include bloating, constipation, indigestion, low energy, fatigue, brain fog, depression, weight gain, chronic pain, infections, allergies, and headaches. In Chapter 4, you can take the "How Toxic Are You?" Quiz to assess the toxic overload in your body. If you have concerns about your liver, there are also blood tests that can tell you how well your liver is functioning. However, such a test cannot show the true extent of your liver's functional capacity. In other words, a slight loss in liver function might not show up in traditional blood screening tests. This type of slowdown is often called a "sluggish liver."

Signs of a sluggish liver are:

- Poor skin tone or flushed facial appearance
- Discoloration of the eyes
- Dark circles
- Yellow-coated tongue
- Acne or breakouts around the nose, cheeks, and chin
- Bitter taste in the mouth

- Headaches
- Moodiness and irritability
- Excessive sweating
- Excessive facial blood vessels
- Red palms and soles, which may also be itchy and inflamed

Although there are several organs of elimination in the body, most health practitioners will agree that the liver is the primary organ of detoxification. It has been said that the length and quality of life depends on proper liver function. Cleansing and detoxification are great for restoring balance in the digestive tract and restoring good liver function. Thus, one of the most important organs to cleanse is the liver. The liver works day and night to cleanse your blood of toxins such as chemicals, poisons, bacteria, and other foreign substances. It is critical to keep it healthy and working at peak performance.

There are so many things we do every day that put extra stress on the liver. Things that make it difficult for the liver to eliminate toxins and break down fats are sugar, artificial sweeteners, alcohol, over-the-counter pain relievers, and medications. The liver has to be very healthy to be able to process these substances that are chemical/foreign or unnatural to the body. When the body is overloaded with these toxins, it just stores them in fat cells. In the DEM System, we will focus heavily on detoxifying and optimizing liver function.

In summary, the liver breaks down everything that enters your body and distinguishes between the nutrients you need to absorb and the dangerous or unnecessary toxic substances that must be filtered out of your blood. It breaks down foods, beverages, prescription medicines, vitamins, even pesticides from foods. But when the liver is clogged and overwhelmed with toxins, it can't do a very effective job of breaking down foods and processing nutrients and fats. So, if you're concerned with managing your weight, remember this important point: The more toxic your body becomes, the more difficulty you'll have losing weight and keeping it off.

Twelve Ways to Detoxify the Body

Detoxifying the body and eliminating toxins can be accomplished through various detoxification methods that we'll discuss in detail below. I would encourage you to pick two or three methods to include as a part of your overall health and wellness goals. When you begin detoxifying the body, you may notice a change for the better in your health and energy levels within a few days; however, for others, it may take a few months. Everyone's toxic overload is different, and many factors come into play, such as your health status, weight, metabolism, age, and genetics. So be patient and remain steadfast throughout the detoxification process.

The twelve best ways to effectively detoxify and cleanse the body are listed below.

1. Colon-cleansing herbs/supplements
2. Colonics
3. Liver-cleansing herbs/supplements
4. Foods that detoxify the body

5. Saunas

6. Bikram yoga

7. Detox foot pads/detox foot bath

8. Alkaline water

9. Body brushing

10. Light physical activity

11. Castor oil packs

12. The Master Cleanse

I have done each one of these detox methods on numerous occasions and perform my personal favorites on a weekly basis. You should think of detoxification as a regular, ongoing activity that will help you stay healthy and slim.

Colon-Cleansing Herbs/Supplements

Colon-cleansing herbs have been used safely for centuries and work a little slower than colonics to detoxify the body but in time achieve good results. They come in the form of powdered or capsule supplements. Their purpose is to force the colon to expel its contents.

A benefit of colon cleansing is the reduction of constipation. A poor diet that deprives someone of essential nutrients can cause the intestinal walls to become lined with a plaque-like substance that is not at all good for health. Colon cleansing not only helps remove the junk from intestinal walls, it also allows waste to pass off more freely. The other noticeable benefit is the elimination of diarrhea. It is a particular condition that is normally caused by toxins, which can also cause problems for the whole process of solidifying the waste.

A very powerful and effective colon cleanser that I've used for overnight results is a magnesium-oxygen supplement. It combines magnesium oxide compounds that have been ozonated and stabilized to release oxygen over twelve hours or more throughout the entire digestive system. The magnesium acts as a vehicle to transport the oxygen throughout the body and has the gentle effect of loosening toxins and acidic waste and transporting them out of the body. Oxygen also supports the growth of friendly bacteria, which is essential for proper digestive and intestinal health.

For intensive colon cleansing, magnesium-oxygen supplements taken for seven to ten days are an effective way to jumpstart a detoxification program. It is safe for regular use and can also be used on a longer-term basis for daily, ongoing detoxification. In contrast to synthetic laxatives, a quality magnesium-oxygen supplement is non-habit-forming and actually strengthens all the organs' functions, making it a safe, long-term option. As always, check with your doctor and be sure to follow the directions on the label. For most people, anywhere from three to five supplements taken at bedtime for seven to ten days will provide an effective colon cleansing. If you experience loose stools or other side effects, simply reduce the dosage and be sure to take just once a day.

Magnesium-oxygen supplements are safe for regular use, but I would recommend they be used only periodically during heavy detoxification and cleansing to help keep the colon clean and increase bowel activity. My favorite brand is Mag07, which has been helpful in my personal journey of cleansing and detoxification. This is also a good alternative for my clients who cannot afford or do not have access to colonics (i.e., colon hydrotherapy). Some clients just rave about its ability to decrease bloating, gas, and constipation. However, for me, it's the detoxification benefits of eliminating impacted toxins and acidic waste from the digestive tract that provides the biggest benefit.

You can also find colon-cleansing products on the Internet or in health-food stores, supermarkets, or pharmacies. They include strong herbal teas, enzymes, powders, or anti-parasite capsules. My two favorite brands of colon-cleansing kits, which involve taking many supplements over a number of days, are Blessed Herbs and Colonix.

Different herbs perform different actions and therefore produce different results, so it's important to know what goal you would like to achieve when choosing your herbal colon-cleansing product. Some work like a laxative to help you eliminate fecal matter and prevent toxic buildup; others kill harmful bacteria and parasites; others soften the stool, add bulk, and improve the function of colon muscles to promote healthy and regular bowel movements. So if you want a product that works strictly as a laxative, you will make a different choice than someone who wants to add bulk and clean out the colon or kill parasites. Please watch the stool to see what comes out. You will be amazed, and possibly disgusted.

Colonics

A colonic, also known as colon hydrotherapy, is a method used to remove waste and impacted fecal matter from the colon. The first modern colonic machine was invented about a hundred years ago. Today, colonic hygienists or colon therapists perform colonics.

Colonics work somewhat like an enema but involve much more water and none of the odors or discomfort. While you lie on a table, a machine or gravity-driven pump slowly flushes up to 20 gallons of water through a tube inserted into the rectum over the course of an hour. After the water is in the colon, the therapist may massage your abdomen. Then the therapist flushes out the fluids and waste through another tube. The therapist may repeat the process. A session may last up to an hour. The therapist may use a variety of water pressures and temperatures.

The average colon weighs up to four pounds, but it is not unusual at all for colon cleansing to flush away as much as ten to twenty pounds of stagnant fecal matter. Your colon can hold a great deal of waste material that, when not eliminated, putrefies, adding to the toxic load of your body. Many people with "potbellies" may actually have several pounds of old, hardened fecal matter lodged within their colons. As a result, the process will actually cause you to experience some immediate weight loss.

It is a common misconception that doing a colonic will cause your body to get rid of all the good and bad bacteria. If you decide to do a colonic, it will rinse out good bacteria in your colon—but just temporarily. After you flush out everything, the good bacteria with the bad, you want to replace the good bacteria, the probiotics. Your body will replenish the good bacteria within twenty-four hours, unless you are extremely unhealthy or weak. However, you should always take a probiotic supplement after a colonic to replenish the good bacteria right away. A good colon therapist will always provide you with probiotics (good bacteria) at the end of your colonics session.

If you choose to research colonics and decide to include them as part of your detoxification process, you probably want to go at least once a week for up to six weeks, particularly when you first begin aggressively detoxifying the body. That is because you are drawing out toxins in the body, and if they are not eliminated quickly, they can cause detox symptoms that become uncomfortable. One rule of thumb as to whether to do a colonic is determined by how frequent your bowel movements are. If your body is managing the toxins and waste well through normal daily bowel movements (one to two per day), then you probably don't need to have a colonic. If your bowel movements are less frequent than once a day, it may be a good idea to do a colonic to get your bowels moving more frequently.

There are no major drawbacks to a properly administered colonic by a trained colon hydrotherapist. You don't need to be concerned about the safety of colonics as long as they're done with a certified colon therapist on a good-quality machine.

Check Your Poop to Evaluate Your Health

Here is another simple way to evaluate your health. As an example, bowel movements (BMs) that are black or reddish indicate potential health problems. Thin BMs suggest that more fiber is needed in the diet or there is some type of imbalance in the digestive tract. If you have chronic constipation and your BMs are rock solid, this may be an indication that your liver is overworked. If you experience chronic constipation or difficult bowel movements for an extended period of time, you should seek medical advice.

Your bowel movements will help you understand what's going on with your body. Healthy bowel movements should:

- Occur two to three times a day and definitely no less than once per day.

- Not have a strong, foul odor.

- Be medium brown in color, shaped like a banana, about the width of a sausage.

- Be 4 to 8 inches long and should enter the water smoothly and slowly fall once it reaches the water.

These guidelines should help you check your poop to constantly evaluate the overall health of your digestive system and toxic overload in your body.

Liver Cleansing Herbs/Supplements

Earlier in this chapter, we discussed how important the liver was to losing weight and staying healthy. The liver is responsible for breaking down and eliminating toxins in the body, as well as breaking down fats in the body. Therefore, it is essential that we cleanse the liver to improve the body's detoxification capabilities and to help the body metabolize and burn fats.

One easy way to cleanse the liver is to take herbs/supplements, such as milk thistle, dandelion root, and burdock. These herbs are all-natural and very effective at liver detoxification. You'll find that many products on the market combine these herbs into one supplement so that you can achieve the best results. As you look for products to help you cleanse your liver, be sure to only use those that are all-natural and gentle on the body. My favorite two liver cleansing supplements are Liver Rescue by Healthforce and Livatone Plus by Dr. Sandra Cabot. Additionally, an inexpensive liver cleansing option is to drink one to two tablespoons of apple cider vinegar in eight ounces of water every morning and night. Do this for two to three weeks or continue until your sluggish liver symptoms have improved. My favorite brand is Bragg Apple Cider Vinegar.

Completing a liver cleanse can be a positive and reju- venating experience and yield numerous health benefits. As you improve liver health, you increase your body's ability to detoxify itself, improve its fat-burning capabilities, and achieve optimum health.

Foods That Detoxify the Body

When you eat natural, organic healthy foods, you keep your insides clean and begin to look radiant despite your age. When you eat more natural, raw foods, you simply look and feel better. Foods and herbs that detoxify and cleanse the body are:

- *Green leafy veggies.* When you are ready to detox your body, fill your refrigerator with kale, wheatgrass, spinach, spirulina, alfalfa, chard, arugula, and other organic leafy greens. These veggies are even better for cleansing the body when they are eaten raw or juiced raw in a juicer. These plants will help give a chloro- phyll-boost to your digestive tract. Chlorophyll rids the body of harmful environmental toxins from smog, heavy metals, herbicides, cleaning products, and pesticides. Green leafy veggies are also high in naturally occurring sulfur and glutathione, which help the liver detoxify harmful chemicals.

- *Onions.* Onions, scallions (green onions), and shallots are sources of sulfur-containing amino acids. According to Patrick Holford and Fiona McDonald Joyce, authors of the book *The 9-Day Liver Detox Diet*, sulfur drives a critical liver-detox pathway known as sulfation. The amino acids present in onions provide the raw materials to make glutathione, a detoxifying compound in the liver. Glutathione detoxifies acetaminophen and caffeine that pass through the organ. These authors recommend eating a small onion, a shallot, or four green onions raw every day to garner the full detoxifying effect. Raw red onions are particularly beneficial as they contain quercetin, a natural anti-inflammatory that enhances liver function.

- *Citrus fruits (grapefruits, lemons, limes, and oranges).* These citrus-filled wonders aid the body in flushing out toxins as well as jumpstarting the digestive tract with enzymatic processes. They also aid the liver in its cleansing processes. To increase detoxification, start each morning with a warm glass of lemon water. Remember, vitamin C is a great detoxification vitamin as it transforms toxins into digestible material.

- *Broccoli sprouts.* Broccoli sprouts are extremely high in antioxidants and can help stimulate the detoxification enzymes in the digestive tract like no other vegetable. The sprouts are actually more effective than the fully grown vegetable.

- *Garlic.* This pungent bulb stimulates the liver to produce detoxification enzymes that help filter out toxic residues in the digestive system. Adding sliced or cooked garlic to any dish will help aid any detox diet.

- *Seeds and nuts.* Incorporate more of the easily digestible seeds and nuts into your diet. These include flaxseed, pumpkin seeds, almonds, walnuts, hemp seeds, sesame seeds, chia seeds, Siberian cedar nuts, and sunflower seeds.

- *Omega-3 oils.* Use hemp oil, avocado oil, olive oil, fish oil, or flaxseed oil while detoxing. These will help lubricate the intestinal walls, allowing the toxins to be absorbed by the oil and eliminated by the body.

- *Beans.* Eat plenty of beans. Beans contain the potent enzyme cholecystokinin, which naturally suppresses your appetite while providing protein to your liver to help detox your body. Add beans to your meals easily by adding them to your salad or just eating them as a side dish.

- *Green Tea.* Packed full of antioxidants, green tea not only washes toxins out of the system through its liquid content, it also contains a special type of antioxidant, called catechins, known to increase liver function.

Saunas

The skin is the largest organ of elimination for the body, and a sauna helps you sweat out toxins from the body. Why I love the sauna is that I'm all about things that have a health benefit while providing a beauty benefit. You can kill two birds with one stone. You release toxins, burn calories, and come out with glowing skin. I personally love getting in the sauna. I had a client that learned about saunas from my teleseminars and found that after using the sauna, her acne cleared up; she was sweating out the toxins instead of letting them clog up her pores.

If you want to know how healthy someone is, sometimes you can just look at his or her skin and tell. If someone has clear, radiant skin, there's a good chance he or she is very healthy; breakouts, puffiness, or dry skin indicate that the body is having some health problems. Experts say that a sauna session can do more to clean, detoxify, and simply "freshen" your skin than anything else.

Benefits of the Sauna:

- *Weight loss.* Burn 300 to 500 calories in fifteen to twenty minutes, almost equivalent to one to two hours of brisk walking or one hour of exercise. Saunas works positively on metabolism, increasing its speed and intensity, which in turn results in weight loss.

- *Elimination of toxins.* Steam saunas induce perspiration, which is how the body purges itself of toxins and impurities. The heat of the steam causes the body's temperature to rise, which can help kill any virus, bacteria, fungus, or parasite in the body.

- *Improved skin.* Steam opens up the pores of the skin, allowing impurities and toxins to flush themselves out of the body. The steam also hydrates and moisturizes the skin, making steam saunas particularly beneficial to people with dry skin.

- *Strengthened immune system.* The steam in a steam

sauna opens up the pores, allowing the skin to sweat out toxins that can cause illness. The high temperature of a steam sauna causes an artificial fever, which sends a "wake-up call" to the immune system and increases an individual's white blood cell count.

- *Relaxed muscles.* The heat from the steam warms and relaxes tense muscles. This relaxation helps to reduce stress levels, revive mental clarity, and improve overall physical and emotional health.

For a steam sauna, you sit in moist heat for fifteen to twenty minutes. Follow that with a quick shower to wash off all of the toxins that have been flushed from your skin and to feel truly refreshed.

Another type of sauna is an infrared sauna, which produces what is known as radiant heat. The heat of an infrared sauna also penetrates more deeply without the discomfort and draining effect often experienced in a conventional steam sauna. An infrared sauna produces two to three times more sweat volume, and due to the lower temperatures used (110 to 130 degrees), it is considered a safer alternative for those at cardiovascular risk. It accelerates the removal of toxic wastes and chemicals that are stored and lodged in the fatty tissues of the body. The sweating caused by deep heat helps eliminate dead skin cells and improve skin tone and elasticity. The heat produced in infrared saunas is extremely helpful for various skin conditions, including acne, eczema, and cellulite. Another benefit of the sauna is that you burn calories. Studies have shown that you can burn 600 calories in thirty minutes in an infrared sauna. Whichever you prefer, steam or infrared sauna, both can be dehydrating, so it is important to hydrate properly before and after a sauna.

A few of my personal tips for using a sauna:

- It is important to try out different types of saunas (steam, infrared, and oxygen steam sauna); you can make appointments at spas to see which type of sauna you like the best.

- You might want to invest in a home steam sauna. I bought one through Amazon.com for about $200, which is a lot cheaper than going to the spa every week.

- Sitting in the sauna one to two times per week is ideal for getting the best results.

- You will need to drink water before and after you get in the sauna. I drink coconut water after my sauna because it is super hydrating.

- If you have heart issues, particularly sensitive skin, or asthma, or if you are pregnant, you should not sit in a sauna until you have checked with your doctor.

Bikram Yoga

I once heard that doing Bikram yoga for detoxification is one of the best ways to rid your body of unwanted wastes and toxins. Now that I have done Bikram yoga, I would definitely agree! During a Bikram yoga class, the body removes toxic waste through the skin via sweat, as your skin is one of the largest waste-disposal systems in the body.

On its own, yoga is already a powerful fitness regimen because you work out every muscle in the body, making them all strong and flexible. In the ninety-minute Bikram yoga class, there are twenty-six poses performed during each session, along with two breathing exercises. The poses are performed in a room with temperatures reaching between 95 and 100 degrees Fahrenheit. At high temperatures, you will begin to sweat profusely, allowing the toxic waste to be removed from the body. This allows your skin to convert toxins that come from various fats into simpler, more water-soluble compounds that can be easily removed. It has been reported that you actually burn 750 to 900 calories in a ninety-minute Bikram yoga session. As an added benefit, you get to learn the techniques of meditation, which can help you relax your mind and alleviate stress. Bikram yoga is an effective means to achieving balance among mind, body, and spirit.

Detox Foot Pads/Detox Foot Bath

Detox foot pads are a quick and easy way to rid the body of toxins. You put the pads on the bottoms of your feet overnight as you sleep. The ingredients in the detox foot pads are said to pull impurities and toxins out of your system during the night while you sleep. In the morning, you remove the pads from your feet and discard them. They are helpful with aches, pains, sore muscles, joint pains, swelling, and bloating.

The detox foot bath (ionic foot bath) works by soaking your feet in a warm saltwater solution made up of many different toxin-drawing ingredients. The ionic activity in the water shoots through your body fat and is supposed to draw the toxins out through the hundreds of pores in your feet. Thirty minutes is the average time for a detox foot bath, which costs a little more than the foot pads ($15 vs. $60 for a detox foot bath). A detox foot bath is said to make joint movement easier in the knees and elbows. It's an alternative medicine option for people who suffer headaches and chronic joint and bone pain. A detox foot bath is very simple and extremely relaxing! If you want to get a detox foot bath, it is typically offered as a spa service under the name of Aqua Chi Foot Bath. For detox foot pads, my favorite brand that I use is BodyRelief Foot Pads, which really helps me with joint aches and pains.

Alkaline Water

Drinking alkaline water (ion water or hydrogen-rich water) detoxifies the body and leaves the skin looking smoother, more elastic, and more youthful. The benefits of drinking alkaline water are detoxification, better hydration, and increased energy. Some brands of alkaline bottled water include Blue Delta and Essentia Water. You can buy a portable alkaline water bottle (e.g., IonPod) that converts regular water to alkaline water or buy an expensive machine that converts the water from your faucet to alkaline water (such as Kangen Water).

It is recommended that you don't drink alkaline water with food or within thirty minutes before or after meals. You also want to build up how much alkaline water your body can handle, beginning with about eight ounces a day. If you drink too much alkaline water too quickly, you will get strong detox symptoms, such as headaches or rashes.

Body Brushing

Body brushing (also known as dry brushing) is done with a

natural boar-bristle brush, which can be found in health food stores, Whole Foods, or Trader Joe's. Dry brushing on a regular basis lightens the burden on the liver by helping to remove excess waste in the body. Dry brushing stimulates the lymphatic system, which is a secondary circulatory system underneath the skin that rids the body of toxic wastes, bacteria, and dead cells. By body brushing, you move the toxins along and out of the body for elimination. By brushing the body from head to toe with the dry brush, focusing on the lymphatic drainage regions, like behind the knee, you'll improve the efficiency of the whole lymphatic system.

Firm, gentle brush strokes across the skin will improve your blood circulation, clean out clogged pores, and enable your body to remove toxins faster. Body brushing removes dead skin layers and encourages cell renewal for smoother skin. If the liver is the fat-burning organ, then the lymph system can be called a fat-processing system. So cleansing the liver and lymphatic system are key to weight loss and diminishing cellulite.

To effectively use the body brush, first remove your clothes. Begin brushing the soles of the feet. Next, brush from the ankles to the calves, concentrating on the area behind the knees, using long upward, firm strokes toward the heart. Then brush from the knees to the groin, the thighs, and the buttocks. If you're a woman, make circular strokes around your thighs and buttocks to help mobilize fat stores, such as cellulite. (Dry brushing actually helps to diminish cellulite.) Then brush the torso, avoiding the breasts. Finally, make long strokes from the wrists to the shoulders and underarms. The entire process should take no more than three to five minutes and will leave your skin feeling totally invigorated. The best times to brush are in the morning before showering or at night before you go to bed.

Light Physical Activity

Just by doing mild or light physical activity, you oxygenate your body to protect it against toxic overload. Simple movements increase the oxygen content of your blood and dissolve and wash out sludge that accumulates in and on your arteries; in other words, it cleanses waste from your bloodstream. For example, as little as thirty minutes of brisk walking can prompt this type of cleansing.

Castor Oil Packs

Castor oil packs are typically used by naturopaths to help stimulate and detoxify the liver. A castor oil pack is placed directly on the skin to increase circulation and to promote elimination and healing of the tissues and organs underneath the skin. It is used to stimulate the liver, relieve pain, increase lymphatic circulation, reduce inflammation, and improve digestion.

Castor oil packs are made by soaking a piece of cotton or wool flannel in castor oil and placing it on the abdomen and especially over the liver. The flannel is covered with a sheet of plastic wrap, and a hot water bottle or heating pad is placed over the plastic to heat the pack. You keep the pack on for thirty to forty-five minutes while in a relaxed position. Rest while the pack is in place but do not fall asleep and leave the heating pad on all night. After removing the pack, cleanse the area with a solution of water and baking soda. Store the pack in a covered container in the refrigerator. Each pack may be reused up to thirty times. It is generally recommended that a castor oil pack be used for three to seven days in one week as a detoxification treatment.

You can place the cloth on the right side of the abdomen to stimulate the liver or directly on inflamed and swollen joints and muscle strains. It can be used on the abdomen to relieve constipation and other digestive disorders and on the lower abdomen in cases of menstrual irregularities and uterine and ovarian cysts. Castor oil should not be taken internally. It should not be applied to broken skin or used during pregnancy, breastfeeding, or during menstrual flow.

The Master Cleanse

The Master Cleanse is an advanced detoxification method, and it's a great way to jumpstart weight loss. It cleans out the accumulated fats in your tissues and liver while purging excess fluid buildup from your system. The Master Cleanse is designed to support all the organs involved in detoxification—the liver, kidney, lungs, lymphatic system, colon, and skin.

Detoxification diets like the Master Cleanse have crossed into the mainstream and are often marketed as a quick and easy way to lose weight. However, the Master Cleanse is not a weight-loss system; rather, it's a way to detoxify and cleanse the body, restoring it to great health. View the Master Cleanse as a stepping-stone to a healthier lifestyle. In fact, if you decide to do the Master Cleanse, once you complete the ten days, you should transition to eating healthier, natural foods so that you do not gain all the weight back.

The Master Cleanse accelerates fat loss from fat-storage areas like the hips, thighs, belly, and buttocks. It will transform your body, with the focus on losing inches as opposed to pounds. However, many people do report losing up to fifteen pounds in ten days. Fat cells shrink as excess toxins stored in them are purged from your body, ensuring that you are losing fat, bloat, and water weight but not muscle.

The first phase requires that you eat no solid foods for ten days. Instead, you ingest a "lemonade" drink that cleanses the body, provides fuel, and prevents hunger. You will take in about 1,000 to 1,200 calories a day. This lighter caloric load allows the body to better metabolize and process toxins and remove them from the body.

The Master Cleanse is not actually a complete fast, as you consume up to 1,200 calories each day, depending upon how much of the lemonade drink you have throughout the day. The detox fast is designed to keep you energized enough to work and enjoy your daily activities. As a matter of fact, since detox fasting increases the body's detoxification capabilities, you may end up experiencing more energy after several days on it.

There are many benefits to the Master Cleanse, such as providing a rest to the digestive system. Your body uses a significant amount of your energy every day in digesting, absorbing, and assimilating your food, so the Master Cleanse gives your digestive tract a chance to rest and repair. This, in turn, gives your overworked liver a chance to catch up on its function of detoxification. During fasting, the cells, tissues, and organs expel accumulated wastes, helping cells heal, repair, and strengthen. The Master Cleanse is helpful because it cleanses the liver, the body's key fat-burning organ, and allows it to rest, improving its ability to break down fats more efficiently and operate at peak performance.

The Master Cleanse provides the added benefit of improving your appearance by deep cleansing every cell in your body; your skin will glow with radiance, and the whites of your eyes will become clearer and whiter and may even sparkle. You will feel and look better than you have in years. Your energy will be supercharged. The Master Cleanse rejuvenates the body physically, mentally, and spiritually.

Some people should *not* do the Master Cleanse. They are:

• People who are undergoing chemotherapy or who have completed chemotherapy within the last six months.

• People who are recovering from major surgery or a severe wound or injury.

• Children in their growing years (under the age of eighteen).

• Pregnant or nursing women. Pregnancy is not a time to detoxify the body but to provide nourishment for the body.

• People allergic to "everything" or who have frequent allergy symptoms.

• The obese (more than seventy pounds overweight).

• People in poor general health.

• People with a multi-year history of taking strong medical or psychiatric drugs.

• Those who use medication for chronic health conditions, such as diabetes, heart disease, high blood pressure, or high cholesterol.

• Anyone with cancer or a terminal illness.

• Anyone with kidney failure or borderline kidney function (best identified by your doctor through blood tests).

If you are able to do the Master Cleanse, I suggest you read two books to provide you with all the detailed instructions to ensure success: *The Master Cleanser* by Stanley Burroughs and *Lose Weight, Have More Energy, and Be Happier in 10 Days* by Peter Glickman.

Ten Ways to Detoxify Your Home

To help minimize toxins in your home and environment, follow these tips:

1. Don't smoke or allow smoking inside your home or car.

2. Leave all shoes at the door as opposed to bringing them into your living quarters.

3. Avoid or air out dry cleaning. Use an organic dry cleaner. If you don't have one near you and feel you must use your local dry cleaner, let your newly dry-cleaned clothes air out in the garage or on the porch for a few days before bringing them into the house.

4. Use unscented laundry detergent and fabric softener.

5. Don't use air fresheners that contain solvents.

6. Replace your furnace filters every six weeks with high-quality pleated filters rated a minimum efficiency reporting value (MERV) of 7-9.

7. Buy an air purifier that has both charcoal and high-efficiency particulate air (HEPA) filters for your bedroom.

8. Use tile flooring or real wood flooring instead of carpeting.

9. Ensure that there is no mold overgrowth anywhere in your home.

10. Install a chlorine filter on your showerhead; this will also help you have softer hair and skin as well.

In Conclusion

If, despite your best efforts, you have still failed when it comes to losing weight and keeping it off, it's most likely because you've missed an important key to losing weight permanently: getting the toxins out of the body. One of my clients sent me a note saying, "Thanks for the great detoxification tips, they are working; I haven't even changed the way I eat, and already I've lost thirteen pounds by your cleansing and detoxification tips." I get this quite often. Once you start cleansing, you become more aware of how your body feels after eating certain foods and drinks. You start paying closer attention to what you eat. You start to recognize what nurtures and nourishes the body and what does not. You begin to let go of emotional toxins along with the physical toxins. You begin to let go of people, places, things, and emotions that are harmful and do not nourish the mind and body.

You've often heard people say, "Calories in, calories out." But from now on, the phrase in your mind should be, "Clean the gut, lose the gut" or "Toxins out, weight off." It is possible to overcome genetics and win the battle of the bulge. It is possible to help your body eliminate toxic wastes that slow down your metabolism, throw off your hormonal balance, and cause you to gain weight.

CHAPTER SIX

Correct Hormonal Imbalances

We all know that fad diets are a thing of the past. The mantra "eat less and exercise more" is ineffective for many people who want to lose weight. We know that the no-carb, low-carb, no-fat, low-fat crazes of the eighties and nineties were hit-or-miss in terms of results. But now, we have better scientific information on one of the more important factors that helps us lose weight: hormonal balance.

Welcome to the world of understanding your hormones, the little messengers that control your appetite, metabolism, and how much weight you gain or lose. Please note that if you are a woman over the age of thirty-five, there are three key sex hormones (estrogen, progesterone, and testosterone) that play a role in weight gain. (For a more detailed discussion on weight gain affecting women over thirty-five, see Chapter 15, "Stop Weight Gain During Perimenopause and Menopause.") It is also important to note that hormonal imbalances affect men as they age as well as women. It is estimated that there are over 32 million men expected to have andropause, or "male menopause." Andropause describes an emotional and physical change related to a decline in hormones that many men experience as they grow older.

It is essential to understand how hormones play a role in maintaining our weight. Hormones control almost every aspect of how we gain and lose weight. Some hormones tell you you're hungry, some tell you you're full; some tell your body what to do with the food that is eaten, whether to use it as fuel for energy or store it as fat, which causes us to gain weight. Hormones are responsible for metabolizing fat. By controlling your hormones, you can control your weight.

Hormones affect how you feel, how you look, and, most important, how you maintain your weight and health. When your hormones are balanced properly, you will have great health, beauty, and vibrancy. When your hormones are imbalanced, you have mood swings, you crave unhealthy foods, and you feel sluggish and lethargic. In this chapter, I will explain which hormones are critical to weight loss, how they work, and how they help you stay slim and healthy.

I once had an unexplained weight gain of thirty pounds, practically overnight, in just a few months. If I ate a Big Mac, I gained a pound by the next day. But today I can easily eat 2,000 calories of nutrient-rich foods a day, without exercising, and still maintain my current weight. None of this would be possible without finely tuned hormones that accelerate my metabolism and cause me to burn fat as opposed to storing fat.

When I was in my late thirties, my hormones began to have a mind of their own and made me feel out of control. If you're like me, you've experienced some of the following:

- Adult acne (skin that breaks out more than when you were a teenager)

- Fatigue and low energy, even when you get a good night's sleep
- Eating less and not losing a single pound
- Skin that's sagging and showing fine lines and wrinkles
- Severe mood swings, even when you're not on your cycle
- Unexplained weight gain of ten, twenty, or thirty pounds for no apparent reason—you haven't changed anything in your diet or lifestyle

I knew that something had changed in my body, but initially I didn't understand the effect my hormones had on my metabolism, weight, moods, health, and well-being. Since then, I've studied cutting-edge research about natural ways to balance my hormones and blood sugar levels to support weight loss. Through reading and research, and my studies as a certified nutritionist and weight-management expert, I learned a great deal about endocrinology, the field of medicine that deals with hormones and glands. I was happy to learn that I was not going crazy and that it was hormonal imbalances that were changing the way I felt and how much weight I gained. It was as if a light was turned on and I could finally see a critical aspect of controlling my weight. The more I talked to others, especially women, I realized I was not alone.

I'm happy to reap the benefits of a stronger metabolism now, but for years my hormones were working against me. I didn't understand much about them years ago, but now I know how to ensure they work in my favor.

Hormones Control Your Appetite

Have you ever thought about what tells your brain when you're hungry or when you're full? One of the major reasons many Americans gain extra weight is that their appetite-control system is out of balance. The various chemical systems and messengers in the body that tell them when they are hungry and when they are full have been disrupted. Rebalancing the chemical hormonal imbalances will get your appetite-control system functioning properly again.

There are certain hormones that balance hunger and fullness in the brain that are key to permanent weight control. If you were never hungry, losing weight would be very easy. If you properly control the hormones that are directly affected by what you eat, you will not be hungry between meals and will have sufficient fuel and energy for the day. This will expedite fat loss.

Feeling hungry is one of the most powerful urges we have. When you feel hungry, everything else is secondary to getting food into your system. This is because the brain becomes desperate to get the energy it needs to function.

There are hormones that control your weight, often called metabolic hormones, brain messenger chemicals called neuropeptides, and messenger molecules of the immune system called cytokines, produced in the fat cells, white blood cells, and liver cells. All of these components work together to communicate to the organs and tissues responsible for managing your weight and keeping you alive. Good communication results in a healthy metabolism. These finely tuned systems determine your health and metabolism. They are what tell you that you are full and to stop eating, making the difference between whether you gain or lose weight.

Let's see how these complex messenger signals work. When your stomach is empty, one of the chemical messengers secretes hormones that tell your body and brain you are hungry. Your brain then prepares the stomach to receive some food. When you eat, the food enters the gut and your body releases yet more hormones, preparing the food for digestion. As the food makes its way into your bloodstream, more messages coordinate your metabolism, telling your pancreas to produce insulin. Your fat cells then sends hormonal messages back to your brain to stop eating, along with signals from your stomach that you are full. Your liver then metabolizes or processes fat and sugar and helps use it for energy or stores the excess as fat.

Your body can't work the way it's supposed to if any one of the hormones is out of sync. You have to be able to naturally optimize how all of your hormones work as opposed to trying to address one at a time. They are too closely integrated to address one; if one is out of sync, then there are already other chemical imbalances in the body. The reason I say "naturally" is because this book doesn't focus on expensive drugs or other dangerous methods but rather addresses the underlying causes of hormonal imbalances, which are our diet (foods we eat), lifestyle (sleep and stress), and environmental factors (toxins and pollutants).

Six Hormones That Affect Weight Gain

There are six hormones that affect weight, and when they are unbalanced, it will be difficult for you to lose weight.

Here is a brief overview of how these six hormones affect weight gain.

Glucagon

Glucagon is a hormone secreted by the pancreas that raises blood glucose levels. It has the opposite effect of insulin, which lowers blood glucose levels. Without adequate levels of glucagon, you will feel hungry and tired because the brain is not getting enough fuel (blood sugar). It is important to balance insulin and glucagon in the body to maintain blood sugar levels. If insulin makes you store fat, then glucagon helps you burn it. It works in the liver to help regulate both blood sugar and fat usage. Eating protein affects the hormone glucagon, which is why eating protein and carbohydrates together is crucial for maintaining stable blood sugar levels.

Cortisol

Cortisol is secreted by the adrenal glands and its primary functions are to increase blood sugar and aid in fat, protein, and carbohydrate metabolism. When you are stressed, your body releases cortisol (also known as the stress hormone). Fat caused by stress (i.e., stress fat) stores in the belly. Studies have shown that when cortisol is released into the bloodstream, you become less sensitive to leptin, the hormone that tells your brain you are full. When this happens, you tend to eat more and begin to crave sugar. That means that your body not only slows down your metabolism when you are stressed out, it actually tells you to consume more food. Cortisol can be very good or very bad. If cortisol is released with high insulin levels and low testosterone, it can store fat; and if it is released with large amounts of testosterone, it enhances fat burning.

Leptin

Leptin is a protein hormone that has a central role in fat metabolism. Leptin is nicknamed the natural appetite suppressant. Leptin controls how hungry you are on a daily basis. When leptin doesn't function properly, it creates an imbalance that results in a slow metabolism, premature aging, and disease. Leptin resistance is a hormonal imbalance that disrupts the body's natural ability to regulate appetite and metabolism. If you become leptin-resistant, you will eat and eat like you're starving. Some people get extremely obese because their bodies never receive the message to stop eating and start burning. Leptin tells your brain when you are full. But when levels are too low, leptin signals your body to store fat. Obviously, you want to keep levels of leptin high in your body, and there are ways to do that naturally. Seafood and fish are known to raise leptin levels because of the omega-3 fatty acids. Omega-3s/fish oil are also available as a supplement.

Thyroid

The thyroid gland is a butterfly-shaped gland located in your neck just below your Adam's apple. Thyroid hormones perform many functions: they help control the amount of oxygen each cell uses, the rate at which the body burns calories, heart rate, body temperature, fertility, digestion, mood, and memory. Thyroid hormones have a profound impact on weight because they regulate how the body burns carbohydrates and fats. Thyroid problems are very common in this country; over 25 million people have some sort of thyroid imbalance. Statistics also show that less than half of them know they have it. When the thyroid is not functioning properly, especially if it becomes under-active, every part of the body is adversely affected. Reduced thyroid activity, or hypothyroidism, causes the metabolic rate to decrease, which greatly affects weight.

Human Growth Hormone (HGH)

HGH is considered to be a "building" hormone because it sends signals to the body to be lean and muscular and work to ensure fat is burned and not stored. HGH is one of the most talked-about hormones of modern times. By now, you should have seen infomercials and products praising the benefits of human growth hormone as the fountain of youth. Our HGH naturally starts to decline in our thirties and forties, and lack of HGH activity promotes weight gain, particularly around the waist and midsection.

Typically, your body will use blood sugar (glucose) for energy before it taps into fat for energy. What HGH does is force your body to draw energy from your fat reserves first, turning your body into a fat-burning machine, even when you're inactive, resting, or even sleeping. HGH is also known to help your body grow new muscle cells, which is particularly good because your body normally stops making muscle cells after your late teens. So, if you do weight or resistance training, HGH will help you get toned muscles. You can naturally boost your HGH levels with certain foods, exercise, and a proper night's rest. Sleep deprivation almost completely destroys HGH production;

it is during deep sleep that the body produces HGH.

Insulin

Insulin is a hormone secreted by the pancreas in response to eating food; its job is to send glucose out of the blood into the tissue cells for use as energy. When excess glucose remains in the blood, insulin levels stay high. Chronically elevated insulin can cause both fat storage and more inflammation in the body. When insulin levels are high, this is a signal to the body to store extra calories as fat and to refrain from burning fat. Because insulin is the hormone most responsible for the obesity epidemic in our country, we will focus on it for the remainder of this chapter.

Insulin Makes You Fat Even If You're Not Diabetic

One of the primary causes of obesity is the excess production of the hormone insulin. Many specialists have stated that it is excess insulin that makes you fat and keeps you fat. Insulin creates fat in the body by taking excess sugar and placing it into fat cells. In order to control your weight, you must control your insulin levels.

Many researchers have found that the majority of people with weight problems produce too much insulin. For most overweight people, insulin is the enemy. The bottom line for most people is that to get rid of fat they have to reduce their insulin levels. If they want to reduce insulin, they have to take away sugar. Sugar (i.e., refined, starchy carbohydrates) stimulates insulin production. And as we've learned from many diet books, reducing carbohydrates is a must. Low-carb diets are initially effective for overweight people because carbohydrates cause the overproduction of insulin, and by cutting out carbs, this overproduction of insulin stops.

However, the key thing to understand is why the body produces too much insulin in the first place. It is due to a hormonal imbalance, which once corrected, will stop the overproduction of insulin in the body. The problem with the low-carb diets is that once you go off those diets, you just gain the weight right back. However, my approach goes further in that it addresses the underlying reason as to why the body is producing too much insulin. Eating fewer carbohydrates helps reduce insulin spikes, but correcting the reason why you produce too much insulin will allow you to address your weight issues once and for all.

Carbohydrates, a key element of the human diet, are abundant in fruits, grains, breads, pastas, cereals, rice, and potatoes. Carbohydrates are the body's primary source of energy. Carbohydrates are broken down during digestion into a sugar known as glucose. Glucose, the simplest sugar, is the only one that the body can use for energy; every one of the body's cells needs glucose in order to function. The amount of glucose in your blood is also called your blood glucose level. A normal glucose level in the blood is 80 to 100 mg/dl.

Now, here's where insulin comes into play. Insulin is a powerful hormone that regulates the glucose levels in the blood. When you have more glucose in your body than your cells need, insulin takes the extra and stores it as fat in the body, allowing your blood glucose levels to return to normal.

Thus, insulin regulates blood glucose levels. But when those insulin levels are too high, it begins storing fat in the body. High insulin levels mean you'll have more body fat, while low insulin levels mean you'll have less body fat. Carbohydrates are the foods that cause these insulin spikes that result in excess fat in the body. When you always have unusually high levels of blood glucose in the body, you have a condition known as diabetes, which is potentially very damaging to the body.

Insulin not only regulates blood sugar levels, it also triggers a biological switch that turns off the production of muscle and turns on the production of fat, particularly around the waist and belly area. That's why you'll often hear insulin called the fat-storage hormone. Insulin also interferes with the breakdown of fat cells, making it even more difficult for your body to lose weight.

What Is Insulin Resistance?

If you have tried different popular diets, counted calories, eaten smaller portions, and exercised but still have been struggling to lose weight no matter what you tried, you may be one of the growing number of people who suffer from a hormone condition known as "insulin resistance." It is believed that 75 percent of Americans have this condition. It is also not uncommon for those who suffer from it to also have other health issues, including high blood pressure, high cholesterol, and sometimes diabetes. If you have "insulin resistance," you can correct both your weight gain and health issues through the DEM System.

Insulin resistance is extremely common: three out of four people have it. But the majority of them don't even know it. I will help you discover if you have insulin resistance and if it's the problem behind your inability to lose weight. You'll be pleased to learn how eating clean and balanced foods help you lose weight if you are insulin resistant. You'll also learn how to combine certain foods to help you lose weight and avoid foods that will cause you to gain weight. You'll see improvements in other health-related issues, including the lowering of high blood pressure and high cholesterol as well.

Insulin resistance, also known as metabolic syndrome, prediabetes, or syndrome X, is a genetic condition that makes it difficult for you to lose weight because your body overreacts to foods that are high in carbohydrates. As a certified nutritionist, I have a great understanding of the science of foods and how foods affect our ability to lose or gain weight. Since I also suffer from insulin resistance, I am personally knowledgeable as to which foods aggravate my condition and cause me to gain weight and feel sluggish and tired. How you eat and what foods you combine are essential to managing insulin resistance and maintaining permanent weight loss.

Each time you eat a high-carbohydrate food or sugar, your blood sugar levels rise, and in response, your body releases insulin to get rid of the excess blood sugar. However, the more your pancreas secretes insulin to control blood sugar, the less sensitive or responsive your body becomes to insulin. In other words, your body becomes resistant to insulin. So then, your body has to secrete even more insulin to lower your blood sugar levels. This creates the condition known as insulin resistance.

Pure sugars, such as sucrose and high-fructose corn

syrups, are digested very quickly, which leads to a rapid increase in blood sugar levels. Additionally, certain carbo-hydrates, such as breads, bagels, muffins, pizza, pasta, and potatoes, are also digested quickly. When blood sugar levels rise very quickly, the body responds with a surge of insulin. This surge leads to excess fat storage in the body while also making you hungrier due to the extreme ups and downs in glucose and insulin levels.

If you are insulin-resistant and eat high-carbohydrate foods, you will produce up to four times more insulin than normal just to be able to bring your blood glucose levels back to normal, healthy levels. I was not surprised to learn that the body can begin storing fat in as little as two hours after eating a high-carbohydrate meal or food, as I had often felt that after a large pasta dinner, I had gained one or two pounds by morning. The good news about the DEM System is that I teach you how to eat clean and bal-anced foods to keep your insulin levels from spiking so that you can lose weight and stay slim.

What Causes Insulin Resistance?

It is believed that insulin resistance is a genetic condition. Some people have higher-than-normal insulin levels and others do not. People who have higher-than-normal insulin levels are considered insulin resistant. This condi-tion causes their body to overreact to carbohydrates by causing higher-than-normal insulin spikes, causing them to get fat faster than people who don't have insulin resistance. The difficult part is that as your body begins to store fat, you become even more insulin resistant, resulting in even more weight gain.

People who consume a great deal of refined, starchy carbohydrates, such as breads, muffins, pasta, potatoes, noodles, and bagels, and sweets, such as cakes, pies, pastries, sodas, sweetened juice, and sugary cereals, have an increased risk of developing insulin resistance. All of these foods cause blood sugar levels to rise and fall rapidly, causing the body to secrete more and more insulin to lower blood sugar levels.

Certain other substances also increase insulin levels, such as caffeine, artificial sweeteners, and nicotine. You may think that your diet soda with an artificial sweetener is relatively harmless because it has no calories and will not raise blood glucose levels, but it will cause insulin levels to rise, contributing to your insulin resistance symptoms. Our goal is to avoid spikes in blood sugar, which trigger insulin release and lead to the storing of fat!

Insulin Resistance Self-Assessment Quiz

To determine if you may have insulin resistance, you can begin by taking the quiz below. Put a check next to every question for which you answer "yes."

Physical Clues

- [ ] Are you at least 30 pounds or more overweight?
- [ ] Do you gain weight even though you eat small portion sizes and small amounts of food?
- [ ] Do you have belly fat, a potbelly, love handles, or weight gain around your waist?
- [ ] Is your waist measurement more than forty inches for men or more than thirty-five inches for women?

☐ Are you of African-American, Hispanic, Native-American, or Asian ancestry?

☐ Do you need to urinate frequently?

☐ Do you experience frequent heartburn or acid reflux?

☐ Do you have skin tags, which are small, painless skin growths on your chest, neck, breast area, groin area, or underarms?

☐ Do you have little to no physical activity on most days?

Emotional and Mental Clues

☐ Do you feel tired after eating, especially in the afternoon, perhaps even feeling the need for a nap?

☐ Do you experience jitteriness, moodiness, or headaches that go away once you eat?

☐ Do you experience foggy thinking or difficulty thinking or concentrating at times?

☐ Do you feel addicted to sodas, candy, and junk food?

☐ Do you feel you eat out of boredom?

☐ Do you feel that you have no willpower when it comes to eating or dieting?

Eating and Diet Clues

☐ Do you crave sweets and carbohydrates, such as pastas and breads?

☐ Do you crave snacks that are salty and crunchy?

☐ For breakfast, do you often eat bagels, croissants, or donuts and coffee?

☐ Do you eat snacks frequently, particularly while watching TV?

☐ Do you drink sodas or sweetened fruit juice every day?

☐ Do you drink beer or liquor at least twice a week?

☐ Do you eat fast foods at least twice per week?

Health or Medical Clues

☐ Do you have a family history of diabetes, high cholesterol, high blood pressure, heart disease, stroke, or obesity or overweight problems?

☐ Have you been diagnosed with either type-2 diabetes or hypoglycemia?

☐ If you are diabetic, do you take a prescription drug to reduce your blood sugar levels?

☐ Have you been diagnosed with a blood clot in your brain, legs, or lungs?

☐ Have you been diagnosed with high uric acid or gout?

☐ Did you grow up around smokers and consume secondhand smoke?

☐ If you're a woman, have you been diagnosed with irregular menstrual periods or polycystic ovarian disease?

If you have marked a check beside fifteen or more questions, then you likely have insulin resistance. Additionally, the more checks you have, the more likely you are to be affected by this condition. To understand additional methods for diagnosing insulin resistance, please see the section below.

Methods to Diagnose Insulin Resistance

Today there is not a consensus among the medical community around the best method to diagnose insulin resistance. However, there are a few practical tests that have been used to help determine if someone is insulin resistant. They include the following:

- *Waist-circumference measurements.* This method is very easy to do. You just use a tape measure to measure your waist circumference. For women, waist measurements of more than thirty-five inches, and for men, more than forty inches, strongly indicate that you have or are at risk for developing insulin resistance.

- *Fasting glucose levels.* This is a blood test that is simple and can often be done at home. This test measures your blood sugar level after you've been fasting (not eating) for several hours. Normal blood sugar levels are between 80 to 100 mg/dl. Levels that are slightly higher, but not high enough to indicate diabetes, may indicate a condition of insulin resistance.

- *Hemoglobin A1C.* Hemoglobin A1C, also called HbA1c, evaluates how blood sugar has damaged proteins in your blood. This test will provide a snapshot of your average blood-glucose levels for the past six weeks. The HbA1c test has certain advantages over a fasting glucose test. Sometimes eating a lot of sugary foods the day before a fasting glucose test will throw off the results of the test. Many practitioners prefer this test because the HbA1c shows average blood sugar in recent weeks, whereas a fasting glucose test just shows it based on what a person has eaten recently. Your doctor can order this test for you. To interpret your test results, a normal HbA1c is 4.5 to 5.7 percent; an HbA1c less than 5 percent is ideal. However, many people suffering from insulin resistance or pre-diabetes have an HbA1c of 5.7 to 6.9 percent, and diabetics have an HbA1c of 7 percent or higher.

Managing Insulin Resistance by Eating "Clean and Balanced" Foods

The bad news is that we cannot change our genetic make-up, and there is no cure for insulin resistance. However, the good news is that insulin resistance can be managed and controlled by eating "clean and balanced foods" and through nutritional supplements that help glucose get inside the cells for energy rather than be stored as fat in the body. There are two nutritional supplements (alpha-lipoic acid and chromium) that are discussed in Chapter 8, which improve insulin function and control your blood sugar levels. Managing insulin resistance not only helps with weight loss, it also prevents numerous other health conditions and diseases.

It will take at least two to three months to reestablish normal insulin sensitivity so that your reaction to carbs won't cause your body to store excess fat. However, most people will experience some improvements within two to three weeks after making the adjustments to their diet and taking the nutritional supplements.

What kind of improvements can you expect to experience? Loss of weight, especially around the abdomen area, improved energy, and fewer carbohydrate and sugar cravings. Additionally, you will want to get your doctor to monitor your lab results every three to four months, as you will likely have improved blood pressure and blood sugar levels. Lower insulin levels help you lose the unwanted body fat as well as reduce your risk of heart disease and diabetes.

Let's describe what "clean and balanced" foods mean. "Clean" foods are primarily natural, whole, raw, or organic—foods that the body can effectively digest and utilize for energy without leaving excess waste or toxins in the body. "Clean" foods include lean proteins, good carbs, and healthy fats. "Balanced" foods mean that you eat protein every time you eat a carbohydrate. So, if you have carbohydrates, you want to always include protein. It is a very simple but effective method for preventing insulin spikes and aiding the body in burning fat.

Why protein every time you eat? Protein counteracts the body's overreaction to carbohydrates, which cause insulin spikes and fat storage. Proteins will also help you feel full longer and thus help prevent overeating and food cravings. Protein will also help you build and maintain muscle mass, and we've learned that muscle naturally burns more calories than fat.

Another way to assist with eating "clean and balanced" foods is to use the glycemic index of foods. Foods with a high glycemic response will raise blood glucose dramatically. Foods with a high glycemic response turn into glucose very quickly and therefore cause a rapid rise in insulin levels. We now know that high spikes and rises in insulin levels cause the body to store fat. However, foods that cause a slower glycemic response will not cause insulin levels to rise and are therefore better for people with insulin resistance. You can always check the glycemic index of foods by going to www.glycemicindex.com. Additionally, there are numerous books and websites available that will list glycemic values for all types of food and beverages. Eating "clean and balanced" foods means eating lean proteins, healthy fats, and more low-glycemic carbs (fruits and veggies), which have little effect on blood sugar and insulin levels and thus prevent the storage of body fat and reduce the risk of diabetes and other health ailments.

Key Factors That Keep Your Hormones Balanced

What causes hormonal imbalance? Too many unhealthy foods, too much stress, and synthetic hormones all cause hormonal imbalances, such as hypothyroid, leptin resistance, and insulin resistance, which all lead to weight gain. But I will give you the tools to retrain your hormones to perform optimally so you can start losing weight and start feeling balanced, happy, and healthy. Additionally, you may want to work with your doctor to run blood tests to determine if you have any specific hormonal imbalances.

The following is a list of ways to keep your hormones balanced.

- *Remove excess toxins from your body.* The endocrine system, which controls hormone production, is especially sensitive to toxins. When the endocrine system is "disrupted" by toxins, hormone imbalances can occur. The chemicals and toxins in the environment send signals to our bodies that make them produce more or less of our hormones than normal. These toxins, which are "endocrine disruptors," confuse the body, causing it to overreact to their signals, disrupting the normal, healthy functioning of the hormonal system. So, getting rid of toxins is key to balancing your hormones.

- *Incorporate healthy, whole foods into your diet.* Whole, fresh, and natural foods repair and restore the normal functioning of hormones. These are the foods that trigger your fat-burning hormones and halt your fat-storing hormones. When you give your body the foods it was designed to utilize, you support your hormones to do what they're meant to do: make your metabolism work for you, not against you. The foods that help restore your body's metabolism and naturally balance your hormones include legumes (beans); alliums (garlic, onions); berries (blackberries, blueberries, raspberries); veggies, especially dark green, leafy veggies (spinach, kale, collards); nuts and seeds (almonds, pecans, sunflower seeds); and whole grains (oats, barley, quinoa).

- *Rebalance your food combinations.* This is where eating protein every time you eat a carbohydrate comes into play. The right "balance" among good carbs, healthy fats, and lean proteins allows you to maintain proper blood sugar levels and sustain your energy throughout the day without hunger or cravings. Instead of counting calories, you'll be eating better-quality foods more often throughout the day. I personally get with eating good food more often! The "food" in the Standard American Diet simply doesn't give our hormones what they need to stay balanced. In Chapter 11, I will teach you how to eat "clean and balanced" foods that assist in keeping your hormones balanced.

- *Lower your stress levels.* You learned earlier that when you are stressed, your body releases a hormone called cortisol, which increases belly fat. Rest, sleep, and relaxation all play a role in lowering the stress in your life. But sometimes you have to "detox" from family and friends who cause you unnecessary stress and strife. People who belittle you and make you feel unworthy should get very little of your time. These people trigger stress and negative emotions in your life. Sometimes they can just say hello, and your stress level increases because you know at the end of that interaction, you will feel low, hurt, or sad. Take steps to minimize the time you spend with these people and find ways to minimize stress in your life.

Chronic hormonal imbalances cause you to gain weight and feel moody and fatigued. You will need to detoxify and cleanse your body—and your kitchen—of the toxic waste that causes you to get fat. You will need to provide your body with healing foods that allow your metabolism to work as a fat-burning machine instead of a fat-storing machine. When your hormones are functioning at their optimal levels, your body is at its peak performance and maintains your healthy, ideal weight.

CHAPTER SEVEN

Speed Up Your Metabolism

Have you tried calorie-counting diets, fat-free diets, small-portions diets, or low-carb diets only to regain every pound you lost while on the diet? Have you tried the weight-loss support meetings and sat next to people who were having success while you looked like you'd been cheating when you really hadn't been?

Have you always felt something was wrong or different about your body, especially as you've watched skinny friends eat twice as much as you and not gain a pound? Well, you were probably right. A combination of factors including aging, stress, hormonal changes, and poor food choices all cause a gradual change in metabolism. You are not lazy, and you do not lack willpower or discipline. Your body simply responds differently to food because you have a sluggish metabolism. I know this because I had a sluggish metabolism that slowed in my late thirties. But through studying to become a certified nutritionist specializing in weight management, I began to learn more about my metabolism and its effect on my weight gain. When I first started rapidly gaining weight, I would limit what I ate. I even tried to work out with a trainer but still gained ten to fifteen more pounds. I continued to gain weight despite following the traditional advice of "eat less and exercise more." But my body did not respond to that advice. So, I knew I needed a different and new approach, and I needed it fast. Thank goodness I found it!

If you find it impossible to lose weight and keep it off, even when you follow all the traditional guidance on dieting and exercising, it is very likely that a sluggish metabolism is one of your problems. It is important to understand how your unique body metabolizes food because that determines how food turns into energy or fat in your body. Most diets don't factor in each individual's metabolism. They focus on dietary changes but don't factor in how your individual metabolism is affecting your weight gain. This is why some people have great success with one diet but others get no results from it at all.

If you have a sluggish metabolism, your body won't respond to traditional diets and weight-loss programs. The traditional diet approach of decreasing calories won't work because weight is determined by your body's response to how foods are processed or metabolized within your body.

Another problem may be that a lot of your weight loss on diets came not from fat but rather muscle, and you need muscle to keep your metabolic engine running effectively. Muscle cells burn fifty times more calories than fat cells. It is important to lose weight in a manner that ensures you will lose fat and minimize muscle loss, which is what we focus on in the DEM System.

How Your Metabolism Affects the Calories You Burn

Metabolism is commonly thought to be a matter of how fast or slowly you burn calories. We often hear people say,

"I can't lose weight because I have a slow metabolism." In general, that is true, but metabolism is much more complex. Metabolism represents all the signals and chemical reactions in your body that regulate your weight and the rate at which you burn calories. A number of factors determine how your metabolism processes food and burns calories, including environment, age, food quality, stress levels, genes, and physical activity. Aging, in particular, has a noticeable impact on metabolism, due to changes in hormone balance. Once you understand what controls your metabolism, you will be able to make changes that will automatically turn your body into a fat-burning machine. When you stop focusing on losing weight and instead on restoring your body to its optimal performance level, the weight loss happens effortlessly and automatically.

Someone with a high metabolic rate is able to burn calories more efficiently than someone with a slower metabolic rate. Any calories that are not burned get converted to fat. Let's take a look at the three main types of calorie burn that happen throughout your day.

Calorie burn #1. The majority of the calorie burn comes from your basal or resting metabolism, which means you burn calories while you're doing absolutely nothing at all. Yes, 60 to 80 percent of your daily calories are burned up by just doing nothing. Whether it's watching TV, sitting in a meeting at work, or sleeping, you are continuing to burn calories. The reason is that your body is always in a constant state of motion. Your heart is beating, blood is pumping through your veins, and your lungs are breathing. This is another reason I say that exercise is not that important to losing weight. Exercise is important for cardio health, but the calories you burn from exercise don't account for the majority of caloric burn happening throughout the day while doing absolutely nothing (your basal metabolism). The calories you burn during your one hour at the gym are relatively insignificant compared to all the calories you burn during the other twenty-three hours in the day. It's more productive to focus on naturally increasing the rate of your resting metabolism—i.e., your caloric burn throughout the day.

Calorie burn #2. The effect of simply eating and digesting your food accounts for about 10 to 15 percent of the calories you burn each day. Studies have shown that during the eating process, your metabolism increases by as much as 30 percent, and this effect lasts up to three hours after you have finished eating. How much caloric burn occurs depends on the type of food you eat. More caloric burn is used to digest protein (25 calories burned for every 100 calories consumed) than to digest fats and carbohydrates (about 10 to 15 calories burned for every 100 calories consumed). That's why the DEM System calls for an appropriate amount of lean, healthy protein.

Calorie burn #3. About 10 to 15 percent of your calorie burn comes from increasing your heart rate, strengthening your muscles, or physical activity, even light physical activity, such as walking up the stairs. In the DEM System, we will discuss ways to "get moving" so that you become more physically active throughout each day even if you don't go to the gym or work out.

How to Avoid Slowing Your Metabolism

One of the greatest myths about weight loss is that for

some people, it is harder to lose weight because they have a genetically slow metabolism. But scientific research shows that this is simply not true. Your metabolic rate is not fixed for life, and, in fact, it can and will change throughout your lifetime.

Yo-yo dieting will alter your metabolism for the worse and make it more difficult to lose weight in the long term. Some of you who are constantly on diets have probably begun to slow your metabolism unknowingly. Here's how this has happened: When someone goes on a diet, the body notices that it is not getting as much food as it used to or as it needs to, so in order to conserve energy, the body slows its metabolic rate. It also begins storing fat reserves to ensure that it will have enough energy throughout the day.

Another problem with endless dieting is that you begin to lose lean muscle mass, which controls your metabolic rate and helps you burn body fat. When the body isn't getting enough food from the diet, it must conserve energy, so the body begins to "eats itself" to get the extra energy it needs. Thus, in addition to slowing your metabolism, you also may be actually losing muscle mass.

Instead of dieting and eating less, you actually want to eat more, when you're hungry, which for most people is every three to four hours. Eating every three to four hours signals your body that you have plenty of food and energy to fuel the body throughout the day, causing the body to speed up metabolism to allow the energy to be used most efficiently.

Your metabolism will naturally slow as you age. It's true!

Your metabolism *does* slow down with age. Starting at about age twenty-five, the average person's metabolism declines between 5 percent and 10 percent per decade. So you will have to work harder and be more deliberate about speeding up your metabolism as you age.

If you're like me and over forty, you probably have blamed your weight gain on your slow or sluggish metabolism. Well, you are correct because as you age, your metabolism tends to slow down. Thus, if your resting metabolic rate is, say, 1,200 calories per day at age forty, it will be around 1,140 at age fifty. So after forty, you may have to make dietary or lifestyle changes just to maintain your current weight.

Compounding things is the reality that, as we age, life gets more hectic and fast-paced, especially if we work or have children or aging parents. This causes us to eat on the run, which means eating fast foods or less healthy foods because that's all we have time for.

Twelve Ways to Boost Your Metabolism

As I said earlier, you definitely have the ability to speed up or slow down your metabolism. Because everyone's body is different, some of the methods to speed up your metabolism will work extremely well, while others not so well. I know for me, drinking green tea gives me a very noticeable boost in my metabolism because I not only burn fat, I also notice less cellulite as well. Pay close attention to your body and how it responds to each metabolism booster. You will want to incorporate as many metabolism boosters as you can, but it's best to not try them all at the same time so that you can figure out which ones are working well and which ones not so well. Then you can continue with the most effective methods on a consistent, regular basis.

Here are twelve easy ways to boost your metabolism to burn more calories:

1. *Just stand up.* A study by Missouri University researchers discovered that inactivity (four hours or more) causes a near shutdown of an enzyme that metabolizes fat and cholesterol. This causes you to store more fat as opposed to the body burning fat. If you are going to be sitting for long periods of time, be sure to stand up once in a while and, if possible, simply walk around the room.

2. *Eat breakfast.* Have a hearty breakfast to rev up your metabolism for the day. Eating a high-protein breakfast wakes up your liver and kicks your metabolism into gear. A high-protein breakfast can increase your metabolic rate by 30 percent for up to twelve hours, which is the calorie-burning equivalent of a three- to five-mile jog. It is important to feed your body every three to four hours and not skip any meals. You especially don't want to skip breakfast. When you skip breakfast, it means your body goes without fuel for about fifteen hours, including the overnight hours. This causes it to automatically store fat over the next twenty-four hours because it thinks it's in starvation mode or a deprived state.

3. *Eat more frequently.* The goal is to not let more than four hours pass without a meal or snack. Yes, ironically, it is important to eat to lose weight! The number of times you eat is important to keep your

metabolism revved up. Every time you eat, you have to burn calories to digest your food, and eating increases your metabolic rate. When more than five hours pass without eating, your body automatically lowers its metabolic rate. In contrast, by eating meals and snacks throughout the day, your body stays at a steady metabolic burn rate that helps you burn calories and fat all day. Remember, we are eating every three or four hours because eating less will slow your metabolism. It sends a signal to your body that it is starving and deprived, causing the body to respond by slowing the metabolic rate and holding on to existing fat reserves in the body. So, eat more. Yes, you can do that!

4. *Don't eat right before going to bed.* Eating before bed is a guaranteed way to slow your metabolism and gain weight. The easy solution is to eat dinner and give yourself at least two to three hours after you eat before you go to sleep. You may even want to eat more lightly at dinner and the heaviest at breakfast. Getting more of your energy from your food earlier in the day helps you lose and maintain weight loss because your body can burn fat throughout the entire day. The fat-burning systems in the body slow, rest, and repair at night while you're sleeping.

5. *Get as much sleep as you need.* One of my favorite ways to boost my metabolism is to get a full eight hours of sleep. When you don't get enough sleep, your energy is low throughout the day. When the body feels tired from a lack of sleep, it seeks to increase energy by consuming food, causing you to crave

more sugar, salt, and fats. In late 2004, for example, researchers showed a strong connection between sleep and the ability to lose weight; the more one sleeps, the better the body can regulate the chemicals that control hunger and appetite. One of these hormones is leptin, which as you'll recall, is responsible for telling your brain that you are full. When functioning normally, it induces fat burning and reduces fat storage.

6. *Get rid of toxins.* Toxins can affect your ability to lose weight by slowing down your metabolism and decreasing your ability to burn fat. As toxins circulate in the body, namely the blood, it slows down your resting metabolic rate. In a study in 1971, the University of Nevada's Division of Biochemistry determined that chemical toxins weakened a special coenzyme that the body needs to burn fat by 20 percent. Toxins (pesticides, food additives, herbicides) interfere with the body's fat-burning process and make it harder to lose fat.

7. *Drink more cold water.* German researchers found that if you drink six cups of cold water a day, it can raise resting metabolism by about 50 calories daily, which in a year can help you to shed about five pounds. This is because it takes more work for the body to heat the water to your body temperature. This is a small thing that can help you lose weight with very little effort. The German researchers also suggest that for up to 90 minutes after drinking cold water, you will keep your metabolism boosted by as much as 24 percent over your average metabolism rate.

8. *Drink caffeinated coffee or tea.* Caffeine is a central nervous system stimulant and can speed up your metabolism by 5 to 8 percent, which helps to burn about 100 to 175 calories a day. This does not mean you should overdo it and drink several cups of coffee. Having one cup of coffee is sufficient, but too many cups of coffee can have adverse side effects. Additionally, green tea, my favorite metabolism booster, is found to provide many health benefits to the body.

9. *Build lean muscle.* As you get older, you will want to maintain as much muscle mass as possible. If you lose muscle mass, your metabolic rate will begin to slow, and you'll burn fewer calories. In fact, one pound of fat burns about two calories a day to maintain itself, whereas one pound of lean muscle mass burns thirty to fifty calories a day to maintain itself. So just by maintaining more muscle mass, you will burn more calories throughout the day and keep your metabolism revved up. Putting on just five to ten pounds of lean muscle mass will speed up your resting metabolism so you will burn more calories even when you're resting.

10. *Eat more fiber.* Research shows that fiber can increase your fat burning by as much as 30 percent. Aim for about 30 grams per day, through either fiber-rich foods or fiber supplements. In fact, there's even a diet whose focus is solely on increasing daily fiber intake as a method to lose weight.

11. *Get moving.* Physical activity of any kind speeds up metabolism, and aerobic exercise gives it a signifi-

cant boost. Also, the higher the intensity of the aerobic exercise, the more it will help your metabolism remain elevated for an extended period of time, so that you continue to burn calories even after you have stopped exercising. In Chapter 12, I discuss ways to "get moving" even if you don't go to the gym.

12. *Spice it up.* One study showed that hot or spicy peppers (chili or cayenne peppers) caused a temporary metabolism boost of about 23 percent. Some people have even purchased cayenne pepper capsules to supplement spicy pepper into their diet daily just to boost their metabolism.

Foods That Speed Up Metabolism

Certain foods are especially effective in speeding up metabolism. They do so in one of three ways: by helping to maintain hormonal balance; by reducing insulin levels, which control fat storage; and by increasing muscle mass (via protein), as muscle burns more calories than fat. These "magic" foods include:

- *Whey or rice protein powder.* Whey protein, which comes from cow's milk, is a complete high-quality protein that speeds up metabolism. If you are a vegetarian, you can use rice protein to accomplish the same thing.

- *Nuts and seeds.* Nuts and seeds are healthy fats that raise the body's metabolism.

- *Green tea.* Studies have shown that green tea is one of the best metabolism boosters you can drink.

- *Beans.* Beans are loaded with fiber, which helps you feel full longer, preventing cravings and binges.

- *Berries.* Berries are loaded with antioxidants and keep your metabolism going strong. Eat them fresh or frozen.

- *Cayenne pepper.* Cayenne pepper is known as a fat burner because it fires up your metabolism. It heats up the body, and the body burns calories when it cools itself down.

- *Vegetables.* Vegetables contain fiber, vitamins, and many essential nutrients that help keep metabolism elevated.

- *Whole-grain cereals.* Cereals such as oatmeal boost the metabolism by keeping insulin levels low after you eat. If you secrete too much insulin, it results in the storage of body fat, which slows down your metabolism.

- *Lean beef, chicken, and turkey.* These are all good sources of lean protein. The more protein you eat, the harder your body has to work to digest it, resulting in more calories burned during the eating process.

- *Salmon, tuna, and sardines.* These fish contain omega-3 fatty acids. French researchers found that men who replaced 6 grams of fat in their diets with 6 grams of fish oil (omega-3 fatty acids) were able to boost their metabolisms and lose an average of two pounds in just twelve weeks. Wild Pacific salmon, in particular, is loaded with omega-3 fats and is a very healthy fish.

Once you begin to boost your metabolism, the weight will come off and stay off permanently. Not only that, but your health will improve as well. You can learn how your body works and how to speed up your metabolism so you burn more calories and fat throughout each day. You'll learn how to get energy from your foods to sustain you all day and keep your metabolism revved up. Weight-related health problems will diminish and, in some cases, even disappear.

CHAPTER EIGHT

Eat Foods That Make You Thin

W hen you eat foods that are primarily natural, whole, raw, or organic, your body can more effectively deal with digesting and utilizing these foods. Healthy foods are recognizable by the body and can be broken down, whereas unnatural foods and ingredients cannot be broken down and will actually cause weight gain, premature aging, and other ailments. The healthiest foods are those that are the easiest for the body to digest—they are effectively broken down and utilized and leave little waste or toxins in the body. In this chapter, we will discuss the following:

- The three foundation foods
- Fiber
- Beverages
- Nutritional supplements

You have probably heard a lot about the need to eat "whole foods." What are whole foods? Whole foods are foods that are fresh and unprocessed and remain almost exactly in the form that they were found in nature. Whole foods include beans, vegetables, whole grains, fruits, nuts, and seeds. As we stated earlier, the quicker your body is able to break down and digest food, the less waste matter it leaves behind that eventually turns into fat cells in the body. Additionally, the longer it takes the body to break food down to digest it, the longer you'll feel full and satisfied throughout the day.

You also hear a lot about organic foods, which are free from chemical preservatives, additives, hormones, pesticides, and antibiotics. Fresh organic foods are far less toxic than highly processed and packaged/frozen foods. Organic foods support good health and help you maintain your ideal weight as well as detoxify the body. Fresh organic fruits, vegetables, whole grains, and meats are best for you. Frozen fruits and vegetables retain many vitamins and often don't contain as many preservatives as packaged and canned foods, but they lack vital enzymes needed for the body to digest them properly. Frozen dinners and canned, boxed, and instant foods are the least healthy options because they often contain sugar, salt, preservatives, and unhealthy fats.

The Three Foundation Foods for Healthy Eating

The three foundation foods for the DEM System are lean proteins, good carbohydrates (carbs), and healthy fats. What you eat is the most important factor in losing weight. You can do all the exercising you want, but if you do not feed your body the necessary foods with the right nutrients that your body requires, then you will hinder your progress toward your weight-loss goals. Knowing what to eat is essential to staying slim. Eating a healthy, well-balanced meal with lean proteins, good carbohydrates, and healthy fats will help you lose weight and keep it off.

What I have learned from counseling my clients is that most people don't know the differences between proteins, carbohydrates, and fats. For instance, many people don't know that fruits and vegetables are carbohydrates. It's important for you to start to think of all foods as either proteins, carbs, or fats. This information is critical to managing your weight long term because each type of food has different hormonal impacts affecting weight gain.

- *Lean proteins.* One of the most effective nutrients for speeding up metabolism and building muscle in the body is protein. Protein boosts the caloric burn while it is being digested and helps to build muscle that also helps burn calories. Examples of lean proteins include eggs, fish, lean poultry, or lean beef (preferably organic and grass- or range-fed meat).

- *Good carbs.* Carbohydrates, particularly those found in their natural form, contain most of the essential nutrients that keep you healthy, give you energy, and turn up your metabolism. Examples include fruit, vegetables, whole grains, beans, nuts, and seeds.

- *Healthy fats.* Healthy fats are the good fats—those that have omega-3 fatty acids that help speed up your metabolism and help your body burn fat more quickly. Examples include fish oil; extra virgin olive oil; cold-pressed plant oils, such as grapeseed oil and sesame oil; nuts and seeds; and coconut.

Lean Proteins

Every one of your body parts, including your blood, skin, organs, enzymes, and muscles, requires protein. High-protein foods are extremely effective for speeding up metabolism naturally. As I explained earlier, the body uses more calories to digest protein than it does to digest carbs or fat. According to a 2006 *Journal of Clinical Nutrition* study, consuming nearly a third of your daily calories as lean protein will increase your metabolism not only during the day, but also when you're sleeping.

Additionally, consuming enough protein helps you preserve lean muscle mass, and the more lean muscle you have, the more calories you burn, even at rest. Eating protein balances your blood-sugar levels so you don't get spikes in energy. It also helps the liver stay metabolically active, especially if you eat it at breakfast, as this helps provide a stable base for energy, mood, and blood sugar throughout the day and evening. For this reason, eating protein at breakfast will help you if you tend to crash in the afternoon.

When choosing protein, you must understand that not all proteins are created equal. You want to be sure you're eating high-quality, lean proteins that have the essential amino acids required to grow, build, and maintain muscle mass, enabling your body to burn more calories throughout the day.

Now that we know that protein can help you lose those unwanted pounds, it's important to eat the right amount and the right kind of proteins to get the health benefits. An average person requires about 50 to 70 grams of protein each day. Five to eight servings of lean protein foods should meet this need. Although a detailed list of lean protein options is provided in Chapter 11, here are some guidelines for selecting good sources of lean protein.

Fish

Fish is one of the healthiest sources of lean protein because it is lower in saturated fat than beef or poultry. Good fish choices include wild salmon, tuna, and sardines. Salmon is extremely healthy and is a good food to eat if you want to shed excess weight. It has an abundance of healthy omega-3 fats, which encourage fat burning. If you have a choice of salmon, always pick the wild-caught kind instead of the cheaper farmed salmon. The most abundant source of wild salmon is found in Alaska, but Canada, California, and a few other states offer it as well. Although both wild and farmed salmon have equivalent levels of omega-3s, compared to wild salmon, farmed salmon is higher in toxins and other chemicals. Wild salmon also is richer in astaxanthin, a very potent antioxidant, anti-inflammatory nutrient popular in the anti-aging industry. Most farmed salmon is fed synthetic astaxanthin, which is inferior to the natural form of this nutrient. Many chefs also use wild salmon because of its superior flavor and texture. Try to eat salmon at least twice a week.

Poultry

Boneless, skinless chicken or turkey breast meat is ideal. Because the skin is loaded with saturated fat, be sure to remove it before cooking. I know the skin adds flavor, but it also adds fat and calories. When choosing poultry, choose white-meat turkey and chicken as often as possible; it is lower in calories than dark meat. The best ways to prepare poultry are roasting, grilling, or baking. Avoid frying because that adds calories.

Beef

Just because you're watching your fat and calorie intake doesn't mean you have to give up beef altogether. If you buy ground beef, get the kind that is 90 percent lean or higher. The label on the package should read "lean" or "extra lean." Choose choice, select, sirloin, flank, top round, London broil, or chuck, which are usually leaner cuts of meat. Avoid meats that say "prime"—these are flavorful but a bit more fatty.

In general, you don't want to eat too much red meat on a weekly basis; however, if you do choose to eat red meats, at least buy meat from grass-fed rather than grain-fed animals. The ranchers who run feedlots typically feed grain to their livestock because it's cheaper and makes their animals fatter and heavier, but the meat from these animals is less nutritious than that from grass-fed animals. Furthermore, grain-fed cattle often have synthetic hormones, antibiotics, and other additives that are passed down to us when we eat their meat. In general, meat from grass-fed animals is lower in fat, cholesterol, and calories. Of course, most supermarket meats are from grain-fed animals, so you may have to go to a whole food or natural grocery store to find the healthier kind. If you are buying poultry or eggs, you'll also want to look for the meat (and eggs) of grass-fed rather than grain-fed animals.

The following health benefits, according to Jo Robinson, author of *Why Grassfed Is Best*, are derived from eating meats from grass-fed as opposed to grain-fed cattle:

- A 6-ounce steak from a grass-fed steer has almost 100 fewer calories than one from a grain-fed animal.

- Meat from grass-fed animals has half the saturated fat of that from grain-fed animals.
- Meat from grass-fed animals has two to six times more omega-3 fats (healthy fats) than that from grain-fed animals.

Beans

Beans, lentils, and peas are also good lean protein sources and have the added benefit of being high in fiber. The protein and fiber content of beans, peas, and lentils will help you feel full longer and prevent overeating. You could easily add them to salads, chili, or soups. Beans and legumes are also carbohydrates but are not as quickly digested as most other carbohydrates, so they function more like high-protein food sources.

Eggs

Eggs received bad press for many years due to cholesterol concerns, but eggs can be included in any healthy diet. If you do have cholesterol concerns, just avoid the yolks, which contain all of the fat and cholesterol. Egg whites are a good high-protein, low-cholesterol choice. An omelet made from one yolk and two egg whites hardly tastes any different from one made from two entire eggs—and it is lower in fat and cholesterol.

As I'll discuss in the next chapter, I am not a fan of dairy products. However, if you do choose to eat or drink dairy products, they should be fat-free or low-fat with no added sugar. This makes unsweetened low-fat or nonfat yogurt or cottage cheese a good protein food source.

Good Carbs

Carbohydrates constitute the biggest group of foods we eat. Those found in their natural form contain most of the essential nutrients that give us energy and fuel our body throughout the day. Unfortunately, most carbs that we eat are the "bad carbs." Foods like sugar, white breads, and white pasta have given carbs a bad rap. But the world of carbs is actually much broader than this. Carbohydrates supply vitamins and minerals, particularly thiamin, niacin, and the powerful antioxidant vitamin E. They are also important sources of fiber, which is an essential nutrient for controlling appetite and making you feel full longer. In short, your body needs carbohydrates not only for energy but also to make serotonin, an important brain chemical that tells you when you are full and no longer hungry.

Unfortunately, most of the carbs that Americans eat are the "bad carbs" found in candy, sweets, junk foods, sodas, fruit juice, sugary cereals, breads, rice, and pasta. The problem with "bad carbs" is that they don't metabolize in our bodies properly, causing insulin spikes, which eventually lead to insulin resistance, causing fat storage in the body.

But did you know fruits and vegetables are also carbohydrates? Nuts, seeds, beans, and whole grains are also carbs. These are all "good" carbs, and if you want to be thin and healthy, you must include these "good" carbs in your diet.

The "good" carbs contain very important ingredients necessary for optimal health and should be a big part of your diet. These include:

126

- Nuts and seeds
- Whole grains
- Beans
- Fruits
- Vegetables

Nuts and seeds. If you are trying to lose weight, add nuts and seeds to your diet. Nuts and seeds provide energy and build stamina because they are such a powerhouse of nutrients. Studies have shown that some nuts and seeds in your diet actually aids in appetite suppression and weight loss. You don't want to eat an entire bag of nuts and seeds because they are calorie-rich, so don't overeat them. Organic, raw nuts and seeds are a better nutritional choice than roasted nuts, which typically are heavy with added oils and salt. A few choices of nuts and seeds include almonds, Brazil nuts, pine nuts, walnuts, macadamia nuts, sesame seeds, and sunflower seeds.

Whole grains. Although whole grains have been recommended because they are high in fiber and rich in vitamin E and B complex, a recent Harvard study published in the *Journal of Clinical Nutrition* showed that whole grains also help you lose weight and prevent weight gain. The Harvard research concluded that women who eat the most whole grains have a 49 percent lower risk of gaining weight and a much lower risk of developing heart disease and diabetes. This research proved that women can lose more weight and maintain their weight loss better than those who eat a lesser amount of whole grains. When you look for whole grains, search for the least-processed, 100-percent-whole-grain cereals, breads, and pasta. As an example, when you eat oatmeal (a whole-grain source), be sure it is rolled oats or oat flakes rather than the instant variety of oatmeals that have added sugar. Healthy whole-grain options include barley, oats, bulgur, corn, millet, quinoa, brown rice, whole wheat, and buckwheat.

Beans. There are many different kinds of beans, including black beans, lentils, red kidney beans, pinto beans, split peas, chickpeas (garbanzo beans), lima beans, and butter beans. If eating beans gives you gas, you can significantly reduce that problem by soaking the beans overnight and pouring out the soaked water before cooking.

Fruits. Fruits provide tremendous health benefits to our bodies by supplying vital amino acids, minerals, and vitamins. Fruit breaks down faster than any other food in our system, leaving us fueled and energized; and because it is a highly cleansing food, it leaves no toxic residue in the body. In fact, fruit dissolves toxic substances and cleanses our tissues, even eliminating old toxic residue in our bodies. In short, fruit is the most life-enhancing food you can eat. Fruits are carbohydrates that are high in fiber and water. Some healthy fruits include blueberries, apples, grapefruit, kiwi, cantaloupe, papaya, blackberries, cherries, and grapes.

Vegetables. In order to be lean, strong, and healthy, you must eat vegetables every day. Studies have shown that those who eat a large variety of vegetables have the least amount of body fat. Green leafy vegetables are especially important because they are low in calories, rich in nutrients, and very high in fiber. This category of vegetables includes kale, spinach, collards, turnip, mustard, and beet greens. Other vegetables include asparagus, broccoli, carrots, eggplant, celery, peppers, cabbage, cauliflower,

Brussels sprouts, and radishes. If you are trying to lose weight, you should limit your intake of starchy vegetables, such as potatoes and corn, as they are higher in calories. Starchy vegetables are also high on the glycemic index, which means they get absorbed into the bloodstream rapidly and cause a surge in insulin levels, leading to excess fat storage in the body. When you reach your desired weight and your weight becomes more stable, you can begin to add the more starchy vegetables to your meals.

You should eat as many fruits and vegetables as possible. A great way to minimize weight gain is to make sure you eat fresh, high-quality, ideally organic fruits and vegetables. One simple way to boost your fruit and vegetable intake is to juice them or drink a green drink daily. A green drink, which we'll discuss later in this chapter, gives you the equivalent of about five servings of vegetables in one drink. I recommend this at least once a day in the morning. I strongly believe that eating vegetables raw, juicing vegetables, or consuming green drinks is key to being slim, radiant, healthy, and energetic.

Buy organic fruits and veggies whenever possible. Certain fruits and veggies, such as strawberries, peaches, pears, nectarines, cherries, grapes, apples, bell peppers, carrots, celery, and greens (such as kale and lettuce), are covered with toxic pesticides and agricultural chemicals. Always look to buy organic when it comes to these fruits and veggies. For other types, such as those with an inedible skin, it is not as critical to buy organic. These include avocados, bananas, papayas, pineapples, watermelon, kiwis, mangoes, onions, sweet corn, and sweet peas. Also lower in pesticides are asparagus, cabbage, and eggplant.

If you can't afford organic fruits and vegetables, wash off the pesticides and waxes as best you can. Waxes are pretty difficult to remove; in fact, they usually can't be removed by simply washing them. You need to purchase special cleansers from health food stores. Be sure to rinse the produce after you scrub off the wax. You can also reduce the toxic content of fruits and vegetables by soaking and scrubbing them in a tub of 10 percent white vinegar and then washing them off with water.

Healthy Fats

Most people believe that low-fat diets are the best way to lose weight, but this is not true. Healthy fats, such as fish oils and coconut oil, not only encourage weight loss but also help you heal many illnesses and ailments. Healthy fats are needed to produce hormones in the body and provide the body with essential fatty acids. However, you should avoid eating large amounts of any fatty foods, as they are high in calories and will cause you to gain weight.

There are essentially three different kinds of fat: healthy fats, bad fats, and ugly fats. I will discuss the good ones here and educate you about the bad and ugly ones in the next chapter.

The healthy fats are the *unsaturated* fats, and they should be included in your diet every day. The best sources of healthy, unsaturated fats are fish, flax oil, fish oil, hemp oil, corn oil, safflower oil, walnuts, sunflower seeds, and pumpkin seeds. An easy way to transition healthy oils into your diet is to use flax oil as a salad dressing, use olive oil for cooking, and take fish oil supplements for added benefit.

You may often hear about a certain type of healthy fat, called omega-3 fatty acids, which are essential unsaturated fats. Healthy omega-3 fats are in nuts and seeds, flaxseeds, pumpkin seeds, walnuts, hazelnuts, pistachios, almonds, Brazil nuts, cashews, and different types of wild fish, including wild salmon, herring, and sardines.

Nuts and seeds are a great healthy snack packed with protein, fiber, and healthy fats. However, if you are over-weight and want to maximize your weight loss, you should limit your intake of nuts and seeds to one serving (one ounce) per day because they are so calorie-rich. However, you should not exclude these healthy fats completely from your diet. As long as you don't overeat nuts and seeds, con-suming them, preferably raw, has been found to promote weight loss and appetite suppression, not weight gain. To understand how many nuts is appropriate for a snack, just think "a handful." A handful (or what you hold in your palm) is generally one ounce. Fill up an empty Altoids box with nuts so you have your handy snack with you at all times. If you prefer to count them out, it would be about forty pistachios, twenty almonds, twenty pecan halves, eighteen macadamia nuts, eighteen cashews, or fifteen wal-nut halves. You don't want to sit in front of the TV and eat an entire bag of nuts while watching your favorite televi-sion show. Healthy eating means avoiding excessive calo-ries and not eating for recreation. Be disciplined about how you snack and be sure to not eat out of boredom.

Nuts are also richer in minerals and vitamins than ani-mal proteins, and nut protein is easily assimilated and does not create uric acid. Raw nuts and seeds are a better nutri-tional choice than roasted nuts, which are usually loaded with added oil and salt. Roasted nuts also lose their freshness more quickly. If you prefer dry-roasted nuts, dry roast your own nuts gently at a low oven temperature, around 150 degrees F, for about ten to fifteen minutes.

Eating Fiber to Lose Weight

If you are trying to lose weight, fiber is known as a miracle nutrient that helps to regulate blood sugar, control hunger, and increase the feeling of fullness (satiety), which will help you lose and maintain your ideal weight for a lifetime. What is fiber? Fiber is the indigestible part of fruits, seeds, vegetables, whole grains, and other edible plants.

Processed foods and refined sugars in our diet have taken the place of fiber-rich fruits and vegetables, leaving us vulnerable to poor health and weight gain. However, eating about 30 grams of fiber per day will help you lose weight, prevent disease, and achieve optimum health. Fiber-rich foods make you feel full, but they are not high-calorie foods, meaning you get to eat a lot of food without consuming a lot of calories. Fiber is a natural appetite suppressant; it curbs your appetite so that you can more easily reduce your caloric intake. Fiber will also improve your digestion and help you maintain bowel regularity.

According to Brenda Watson, author of *The Fiber35 Diet: Nature's Weight Loss Secret*, for every gram of fiber you eat, you can potentially eliminate seven calories. This means that if you consume 35 grams of fiber daily, you will burn 245 extra calories a day.

There are two basic types of fiber—soluble and insoluble.

Soluble fiber dissolves and breaks down in water, forming a thick gel. Some food sources of soluble fiber include apples, oranges, peaches, nuts, barley, beets, carrots, cranberries, lentils, oats, bran, and peas. Soluble fiber slows the absorption of food after meals and thus helps regulate blood sugar and insulin levels, reducing fat storage in the body. It also removes unwanted toxins, lowers cholesterol, and reduces the risk of heart disease and gallstones.

Insoluble fiber (also known as roughage) does not dissolve in water or break down in your digestive system. Insoluble fiber passes through the gastrointestinal tract almost intact. Some food sources of insoluble fiber include green leafy vegetables, seeds and nuts, fruit skins, potato skins, vegetable skins, wheat bran, and whole grains. Insoluble fiber not only promotes weight loss and relieves constipation, but it also assists in the removal of cancer-causing substances from the colon wall. It helps to prevent the formation of gallstones by binding with bile acids and removing cholesterol before stones can form, thus they are especially beneficial to people with diabetes or colon cancer.

You will want to consume both soluble and insoluble fiber because each type provides benefits to the body. Many health organizations recommend that people consume 20 to 35 grams of fiber per day, not to exceed 50 grams. To support weight-loss efforts and improve colon and digestive health, I recommend a fiber intake of a minimum of 30 grams per day. The average American consumes only 10 to 15 grams of fiber daily.

If you're increasing your fiber intake, it is important to drink plenty of water to avoid constipation. A good rule of thumb is to drink half your body weight in ounces of water daily. To determine how much this is, just divide your body weight (in pounds) by two and drink that number of ounces of water per day. As an example, if you weigh 140 pounds, then you want to drink 70 ounces (about nine, 8-oz glasses) of water daily.

The best way to get more fiber in your diet is through foods high in fiber. A few high-fiber food choices are:

- 1 cup bran cereal (20g)
- 1 cup cooked black beans (14g)
- 1 cup red cooked lentil beans (13g)
- 1 cup cooked kidney beans (12g)
- 1 medium avocado (12g)
- 1 cup oats (12g)
- 1 cup cooked peas (9g)
- 1 cup cooked lima beans (9g)
- 1 cup brown rice (8g)
- 1 cup cooked kale (7g)
- 3 tablespoons flaxseeds (7g)
- 1 cup raspberries (6g)
- 1/2 cup sunflower seeds (6g)
- 1 medium apple (5g)
- 1 medium pear (5g)
- 1 cup cooked broccoli (5g)
- 1 cup cooked carrots (5g)
- 1 medium baked potato or sweet potato (5g)
- 1 cup blueberries (4g)

- 1 cup strawberries (4g)
- 1 medium banana (4g)
- 1 ounce of almonds (4g)
- 1 cup cooked spinach (4g)
- 3 cups of air-popped popcorn (4g)
- 1 ounce of walnuts or pistachio nuts (3g)

If you don't get enough fiber in your diet, you might want to try supplements. I have personally used psyllium but had a lot of trouble with gas, bloating, and constipation. I recommend acacia, flax, or oat fibers as a better alternative for a fiber supplement. In addition to fiber supplements, you can eat fiber bars or drink fiber shakes to increase your daily fiber intake.

Beverages That Help You Stay Slim and Healthy

Now we want to focus on the best drinks and beverages that help us lose weight and stay healthy. The best choices are the following:

- Water
- Green tea
- Fresh-squeezed juices
- Coconut water
- Non-dairy milk

Water. The most important thing to drink for weight loss and good health is water! On average, your body is 60 to 70 percent water, with about two-thirds of it in your cells and the rest in your blood and body fluids. Therefore, water is essential to a healthy, functioning body. Water flushes out toxins and supports every metabolic process in the body, carrying toxins and waste away from cells to the kidneys to be removed from the body.

The funny thing is that drinking too little water every day actually causes your body to retain water. The kidneys require an adequate amount of water to flush waste from the body. When the body is lacking water, the kidneys begin to hoard water and the lymphatic system becomes sluggish. You have to keep your body well hydrated. You want to drink plenty of water throughout the day. Drink at least half your body weight in ounces every day. To determine if you are getting enough water and are well hydrated, look at your urine. If it is yellow, you're dehydrated and need to drink more water. The goal is to get your urine as clear in color as possible.

Water can also help minimize cravings. At times, you may feel as though you are craving certain foods, but in actuality, you are just dehydrated. So, anytime you crave sweets, drink some water first. You may find that the craving goes away after drinking water. As it relates to detoxification, an even better type of water is alkaline water. At a minimum, you should drink spring or filtered water (at least half your body weight in ounces), but for truly beautiful, hydrated skin, try alkaline water. Alkaline water detoxifies the body, leaving the skin looking smoother and more elastic and restoring it to a more youthful state. Alkaline water is known for hydrating the skin and keeping the inner body balanced and clean. If you decide to try alkaline water, start out with just a little at first to avoid strong detox symptoms. We discuss alkaline water as a detox method in Chapter 5.

Green Tea. Green tea has tremendous health benefits. It is one of the few caffeine drinks that I strongly recommend. In fact, it is an integral part of the DEM System. Green tea is particularly helpful with reducing body fat and weight, stimulating digestion, and preventing high blood pressure. It has been shown to be twenty times more effective in slowing the aging process than vitamin E because of its strong antioxidant capacity. The vitamin C content of green tea is four times higher than that of lemon juice. There are many wonderful benefits of drinking green tea, but as far as weight loss goes, it simply helps the body burn fat faster and more efficiently.

Green tea is better than black tea or coffee because its caffeine works in a different way. Green tea makes the body's own energy use more efficient, thereby improving your vitality and stamina without your having to experience the up-and-down effect typically experienced with caffeine. This is due to the large amounts of tannins in green tea that ensure that the caffeine is taken to the brain in only small amounts, which harmonizes the energies in the body.

Green tea is very high in antioxidants, but since it does contain caffeine, don't drink it too late in the day or it can interfere with sleep. I strongly recommend that you enjoy green tea (either hot or iced tea) in the morning and for lunch. For detoxification purposes, I recommend one to two cups a day. If you prefer, you may take one green tea capsule two to three times a day instead. My favorite brand is Wu-Long Chinese Slimming Tea.

Just a quick aside about caffeine: About half the research shows caffeine from coffee and tea to be beneficial, and about half suggests it has detrimental effects on the body. I'm with the half that says it can be beneficial and can improve the fat-burning process. Thus, I recommend drinking some caffeine drinks like green tea or coffee in moderation as a part of the DEM System.

Fresh-Squeezed Juices. Fresh-squeezed juices, as opposed to store-bought juices that have additives and sugar, are also very important to your health. Fresh fruits and vegetables are extremely high in enzymes. Enzymes are actually organic catalysts that increase the rate at which food is broken down and absorbed by the body. However, these enzymes are destroyed during cooking and processing, as well as in bottled and packaged juices, so try to eat them fresh or juice them whenever possible. Fresh juice contains living digestive enzymes that are important in breaking down foods in the digestive tract. This preserves your body's own digestive enzymes, giving your digestive system a much-needed rest so that it can repair, recuperate, and rejuvenate. Additionally, fresh juices are rich in phytonutrients, which are important plant-derived nutrients that contain antioxidants that slow the aging process.

Coconut Water. Water or juice from young coconuts is a super-hydrating kind of water that is not only delicious but also rich in minerals, especially potassium. It has almost twice as much potassium as a banana. Drinking it is an excellent way to replace electrolytes after a heavy workout or simply to hydrate the body on a hot day. Many athletes and runners drink coconut water instead of sports drinks like Gatorade. It is fat- and cholesterol-free and low in calories, with positive effects on circulation, body temperature, heart function, and blood pressure.

Coconut water is simply an outstanding beverage for so many reasons. It is my personal favorite these days. In tropical regions, it has been used for centuries as a health and beauty aid because it naturally hydrates the skin. It has a natural balance of sodium, potassium, calcium, and magnesium, making it a healthy drink for hydrating and replacing electrolytes in the body. It is low in calories and has been shown to have antiviral and antifungal properties. The brands I enjoy the most are Vita Coco and O.N.E. Coconut Water.

Non-Dairy Milk. As I'll discuss in the next chapter, there are many reasons to give up cow's milk (dairy), but milk is an important part of a healthy diet. The goal should be to drink healthier milk options. Dairy products made from the milk of goats and sheep are better than those made from cow's milk, particularly if they are raw. The natural enzymes in goat's milk are far closer to those in humans, so we're able to digest goat's milk significantly better. Sheep's milk is the next best choice. There are also non-dairy milk options, such as almond, rice, hemp, or soy milk (all unsweetened). If you still decide to consume products made with cow's milk, buy organic and no-fat or low-fat brands because they are more nutritious.

Nutritional Supplements

No matter how well we eat, it is likely that there will be some nutrients we just don't get quite enough of. Therefore, we should consume high-quality nutritional supplements. Supplements help you maintain your weight, achieve optimal health, fight disease, and slow the aging process. As it relates to weight loss, I recommend nutritional supplements that will help you lose body fat, preserve muscle mass, and regulate levels of blood sugar and insulin, which are critical for maintaining a healthy, slim body. Scientific research has proven that various supplements can help the body better metabolize fats, reduce the inflammation coming from fat cells, and fill in nutritional gaps and deficiencies. The supplements I recommend go beyond the typical multivitamins. These recommended supplements, combined with dietary changes, are your secret weapons against excess fat in the body. Supplements are a part of the DEM System for maintaining good health as you age.

What I discuss in this chapter is a general overview of supplements to provide basic knowledge that you can then take to your physician and local health food store to get specifics on dosage or on how much of a given supplement to take given your current health. Where possible, I will provide my suggestions, but as always, consult your doctor prior to starting any new diet, supplement, or exercise regimen. These supplements can help support detoxification, strengthen the immune system, balance hormones, protect against degenerative diseases, and promote weight loss. Supplements recommended in the DEM System include the following:

- Green drinks
- Fiber
- Fish oil (omega-3 fatty acids)
- Protein drinks
- Antioxidants
- Probiotics

- Vitamin C
- Digestive enzymes
- Alpha-lipoic acid or R-lipoic acid *(for those who are insulin-resistant only)*
- Chromium *(for those who are insulin-resistant only)*

Please note that these supplements do not have to be taken individually. Many are found in multivitamins or in green drinks. As an example, a product called Green Vibrance provides probiotics, digestive enzymes, antioxidants, and fiber. Additionally, the protein drink I use by Rainbow Light, Acai Berry Blast Protein Energizer, contains sufficient quantities of protein, digestives enzymes, antioxidants, and fiber.

Green Drinks. One of the most important supplements I include in the DEM System is nicknamed the "green drink" because it is derived primarily from green leafy vegetables, the same greens that feed some of the strongest, biggest animals on the planet, such as cows, horses, and oxen. Green drinks help you detoxify and cleanse your system, lose weight, have more energy, and make the body more alkaline. When you drink them, the nutrients in them get to the cells very quickly and give the body a real boost.

The green drink I recommend is a high-density nutrient powder (Vitamineral Green) primarily composed of greens including kale, spinach, alfalfa, barley grass, wheatgrass, broccoli, and many others. These greens are harvested at their peak, dried, and lightly processed into powders. This innovative process preserves most of their vitamins, minerals, nutrients, phytochemicals, and enzymes. You simply mix a scoop of the green powder with water or juice, drink it down, and voilà! You just drank five servings of fruits and veggies! I can get extremely busy some days and can't trust that I will eat enough fruits and veggies, so this ensures that I'm covered even before I leave home. When I travel, I have individual packets of my green drink to carry with me on the road. I never leave home without my green drink! Another great green drink option is made by Green Vibrance; it also contains green leafy vegetables and provides probiotics, digestive enzymes, and antioxidants. If you want to begin by adding only one recommended nutritional supplement into your diet, it should be the green drink.

Fiber. In the DEM System, I recommend that you get at least 30 grams of fiber per day. If you are unable to get 30 grams a day of fiber from your food, there are a few convenient supplement options.

- *Chewable fiber wafers.* Try eating a couple of acacia-based chewable fiber wafers. Ask your local health food store for help in finding these.

- *Clear fiber powder.* Clear, tasteless, zero-calorie acacia fiber can be sprinkled on your food to enhance the fiber content without altering the taste of your meals. One of my favorite brands is called Fiber35 Diet Sprinkle Fiber by Fiber35 Diet.

- *Shakes.* Look for shakes that have at least 10 grams of fiber (from acacia) per serving and a decent amount of whey protein (around 20 grams) from a rich source, as well as a variety of important vitamins, minerals, and enzymes to improve digestion. Avoid shakes that contain artificial sugar substitutes. A natural sweetener like stevia is best.

- *Bars.* Look for high-fiber bars that contain about 10 grams of fiber (6 soluble; 4 insoluble) from oat fiber, gum acacia, and milled flaxseed, and 10 grams of protein from whey protein concentrate. Look for a bar that is sweetened with dates, raisins, and stevia or agave syrup.

Fish Oil (Omega-3 Fatty Acids). Supplementing your diet through fish oil helps eliminate excess fat while also rejuvenating the cells in the body. Taking a good-quality fish oil supplement will provide you with the necessary omega-3 fatty acids you need to burn stored fat and maintain optimum health. A high-quality fish oil supplement supplies a concentrated amount of the two important omega-3 fatty acids: EPA and DHA. Fish oil/cod liver oil (ultra-refined EPA/DHA concentrates) is considered a wonder drug for its amazing health benefits. Many people take liquid fish oil instead of capsules, particularly if they want a higher dosage of EPA and DHA. If you do use liquid fish oil, always keep it in the refrigerator to prevent oxidation and to preserve its taste. One of my favorite brands is made by Carlson Labs—I like its quality and light lemon taste.

Protein Drinks. One quick and easy way to ensure you get more protein in your diet is to take a protein powder supplement. Supplementing protein in your diet should help you stay slim, maintain muscle mass, and slow aging. Whey protein (cow's milk) is a high-quality, complete protein source. However, a non-dairy rice protein will also provide benefits for those who want to stay away from dairy. Protein is essential for weight loss because your body uses more energy to digest protein than other foods so it helps you burn more calories. It also helps to slow down the absorption of glucose in the bloodstream, reducing insulin levels, making it easier for the body to burn fat and decrease hunger between meals. Protein also preserves lean muscle tissue, and by maintaining muscle mass in the body, you keep your metabolism higher, which will naturally burn more calories.

Antioxidants. Taking an antioxidant supplement will help your body repair cellular damage. Antioxidants work to sweep up dangerous free radicals that can interfere with cellular function. Two more power hitters in the antioxidants are L-carnitine and Coenzyme Q10. L-carnitine is an amino acid that ushers fats through the cells to the mitochondria where they can be used for fuel. The food with the highest concentration of L-carnitine is avocado. The mitochondria also need CoQ10 for proper functioning. This wonderful nutrient has proved its worth in cases of high blood pressure and congestive heart failure (a definite mitochondrial malfunction).

Probiotics. Probiotic supplements help keep a healthy balance of beneficial bacteria in your digestive tract. There are 500 different species of bacteria in the digestive tract; 80 percent are good bacteria and 20 percent are bad bacteria. Good bacteria are critical to your body's ability to deflect incoming toxins so they don't cause overgrowth or imbalance in the digestive tract. The two most plentiful probiotics are lactobacillus, which are primarily found living in the small intestine, and bifidobacterium, most prevalent in your large intestine. When selecting a probiotic supplement, choose a high-potency formula with significant amounts of both bifidobacterium and lactobacillus (culture counts should be in the billions). I recommend taking a good probiotic every day to help maintain a healthy digestive environment in the gut (colon).

When we take antibiotics, many of the body's beneficial bacteria can be killed, which throws off the balance, causing bad bacteria to grow out of control. If you have had repeated rounds of antibiotics to treat illnesses, you could be at risk for developing an overgrowth of intestinal bacteria. Bad bacteria produce endotoxins, which may be as toxic as chemical pesticides or other toxic substances.

Although there are yogurt products that are marketed to promote good, healthy bacteria, most of them contain added sugars and are not prepared in a way that allows the most beneficial bacteria to thrive in your digestive track. So adding yogurt to your diet to get more probiotics is not a bad idea, but I believe that a high-quality probiotic supplement, like PB8, Culturelle, or Ultimate Flora, is most effective.

Vitamin C. Vitamin C is vital for the proper functioning of white blood cells, which fight off the invading bacteria and viruses that lead to colds and flu. Vitamin C also improves the functioning of the enzymes in the liver, helping to eliminate toxins. Vitamin C helps with detoxification and inflammation. Many health practitioners recommend taking 500 to 1,000 mg of buffered ascorbic acid (vitamin C) powder or capsules daily. Personally, I've been taking about 1,000 milligrams of vitamin C for the past ten years with no issues or side effects. I think this is one of the reasons I've gone from getting four to five colds per year to about one per year.

Digestive Enzymes. Enzymes break down foods during the digestive process by splitting apart the bonds that hold nutrients together. Enzymes are normally present in raw foods, but many processed and packaged foods are depleted of their natural enzymes through cooking and processing. If the body is lacking essential enzymes needed for proper digestion, the body may not be able to completely break down foods and allow the body to absorb their nutrients. When enzymes in food are destroyed, the digestive organs have to work harder to break down and process that food. So you will want to supplement your diet with digestive enzymes that contain protease, amylase, lipase, and cellulase, which can assist and speed up digestion and the body's absorption of nutrients. After taking them, you will immediately begin to experience less bloating and gas.

Nutritional Supplements that Improve Insulin Function and Control Your Blood Sugar. In Chapter 6, we discussed how insulin causes weight gain. In this section, I recommend nutritional supplements that have been scientifically proven to lower blood sugar levels, improve insulin function, and reduce appetite and cravings. These nutritional supplements are not weight loss pills, but if you have insulin resistance, because they work to control your blood sugar and insulin levels, they will cause your body to burn fat and lose weight. If you follow the dietary changes outlined in this book, combined with the recommended nutritional supplements, you will begin to burn fat and become naturally thin.

Alpha-lipoic Acid or R-lipoic Acid. Alpha-lipoic acid

improves insulin function and can gradually decrease blood sugar levels, which helps the body to burn fat. Animal research studies have found that alpha-lipoic acid can reduce appetite, speed up metabolism, and promote weight loss. In addition to being a powerful antioxidant and anti-inflammatory nutrient, alpha lipoic acid increases the body's ability to take glucose into the cells. This nutrient works synergistically to better regulate blood sugar and insulin levels. R-lipoic acid is a type of lipoic acid that is chemically identical to the one found in nature. R-lipoic acid is more expensive than alpha-lipoic acid, but it can be more effective because it's a more biologically active compound.

You can try 100 mg of alpha-lipoic acid or R-lipoic acid about fifteen minutes before each meal, three times a day. However, if you are a diabetic, you can take 200 mg before each meal, three times a day. One of my favorite brands is a product called Insulow (www.insulow.com). This product combines R-lipoic acid with biotin, both important nutrients for managing insulin resistance and controlling diabetes. Biotin plays a crucial role in managing insulin and blood sugar and is a good supplement to take combined with either chromium or alpha-lipoic-acid or R-lipoic acid. More information on Insulow is available at www.insulow.com. Another one of my favorite brands that is very popular is Doctor's Best Stabilized R-Lipoic Acid.

Chromium. Chromium is a mineral found in the body in trace amounts. Research has shown that chromium supplementation has the ability to even out blood sugar levels while enhancing the body's fat-burning metabolism. Chromium is also known to be helpful in suppressing appetite and cravings. Taking chromium supplements may help control carbohydrate cravings and improve insulin function and glucose metabolism. Research studies have shown that many people with insulin resistance and diabetes have chromium deficiencies; thus, taking chromium supplements can help improve blood glucose levels. Taking chromium supplements in conjunction with eating a healthy diet and engaging in moderate physical activity can result in an outstanding degree of fat burning and weight loss.

There are two leading types of chromium supplements: chromium picolinate and chromium polynicotinate. With the chromium polynicotinate supplement, chromium is bound to a form of the B vitamin, niacin. In the picolinate supplement, chromium is combined with the amino acid tryptophan. There is conflicting information about which type is most effective. Studies have shown that while both types of supplements are safe, chromium polynicotinate is more easily absorbed by the body. There is also more research indicating that chromium polynicotinate promotes fat loss but preserves muscle mass.

I have used both types and, for me, chromium picolinate has been much more effective at fat burning and weight loss. However, you should do your research and consult with your doctor to choose which type may be best for you if you suffer from insulin resistance or diabetes. Recommended dosages include 200 to 400 micrograms, three times daily, about fifteen minutes before each meal.

This DEM System is the start of a whole new lifestyle. The end goal is to allow you to lose weight, restore your health, and help you transition into a healthy lifestyle of eating and living.

CHAPTER NINE

Avoid Foods That Make You Fat

Simply put, certain foods cause you to gain weight more than others do, and these items should be minimized or avoided altogether. The foods listed in this chapter have the biggest impact on creating excessive fat in the body as well as poor health.

Sugar

Sugars include refined white sugar, brown sugar, and high-fructose corn syrup. When you eat sugar, you trigger a vicious cycle of sugar cravings, increased insulin production, increased appetite, more sugar intake, and more insulin production, until you are in a cycle of craving, binging, and crashing all day long. Eventually, this leads to insulin resistance, which is a major contributor to weight gain and rapid aging.

Examples of foods containing lots of sugar include cakes, pies, candy, barbecue sauce, breakfast cereals, cookies, donuts, fruit punch, fruit juices, ice cream, jellies, pudding, popsicles, sodas, and yogurts with added fruit. Just read the label and look for sugar in the list of ingredients. As a general guideline, try to avoid products that have more than 5 grams of sugar per serving.

Salt

Many people are aware of the health-related issues, such as high blood pressure and cardiovascular disease, that result from too much salt in their diet. But most people don't realize how salt contributes to weight gain. Salt wreaks havoc on your waistline. A 2007 study published in *Obesity Research* showed that high-salt diets are directly associated with more fat cells in the body, and even worse, that salt makes fat cells denser and thicker.

When you eat too much salt, your kidneys have to work overtime to excrete the excess. The body can best handle only about 1,400 to 2,500 mg per day, but today most people consume 4,500 to 6,000 mg of salt per day. If the kidneys become unable to excrete all the excess, the salt begins to build up in the tissues and damage cells. When your body has damaged cells, other bodily functions suffer, including the ability to burn fat. A high-salt diet also hardens the arteries, which makes it difficult for oxygen to get to your cells. When you get less oxygen into your cells, you will have a less-efficient metabolism, slowing your ability to burn fat.

A high-salt diet makes you retain water and become bloated. Even if you lose body fat, you will remain bloated; you will still look and feel puffy and heavy. Salt attracts and holds water, increasing blood volume and making your body expand and become bigger and thicker. The retention of extra water and fluid results in major bloating. Even after eating a meal high in salt or a salty snack, you'll notice how your stomach begins to look bloated and bigger. Many people with a high-salt diet are carrying around five to ten pounds of extra water weight. When you eat salty snacks,

you become thirstier and hungrier and end up overeating—all things you don't want to occur when you're trying
to lose weight.

Trans Fats

There are three types of fats: healthy fats (discussed in the
previous chapter), bad fats (discussed a little later in this
chapter in the section titled "Saturated Fats"), and ugly
fats—trans fats, also labeled on products as hydrogenated
oils. These manmade fats are the worst of all—considered
by many to be toxic. Your body cannot properly digest
trans fats, and they negatively impact your weight and
health. They are found in fried foods like potato chips,
french fries, and onion rings, and, unfortunately, in virtually every commercially packaged or baked good, including
cookies, pastries, donuts, and crackers, because they don't
spoil quickly and help to extend the shelf life of these products. Eating trans fats is like eating plastic and is very bad
for one's health, yet modern Americans consume them in
large quantities, often without the slightest awareness of
what they are doing. Trans fats disrupt metabolism, cause
weight gain, and increase the risk of diabetes, heart disease,
inflammation, and cancer.

One Harvard study found that getting just 3 percent
of daily calories from trans fats (about 7 to 8 grams of
trans fat) increases your risk of heart disease by 50 percent.
And given that the average person has about 4 to 10 grams
of trans fats in his or her diet, it is no wonder heart disease
is such a major killer in modern times. Learn to identify
trans fats in foods. Read the labels on all food products
before you buy them, and avoid products whose labels

contains the words *trans fat, hydrogenated,* and *partially hydrogenated.*

Saturated Fats

Saturated fats are found in red meat and many dairy products like whole milk, cheese, and butter. Eating a lot of saturated fat can increase cholesterol in your blood and lead to heart attack or stroke. Consumption of these fats should be limited or avoided altogether if possible. To eat less saturated fat, be sure to eat lean meat or skinless poultry, or at least trim the fat before you cook it. You can also eat fewer pastries, cakes, and biscuits—in other words, baked goods that contain butter and/or milk are also high in saturated fats and should be avoided.

White Flour

White flour, commonly found in many desserts and pastas, contributes to weight gain. Don't let the name "wheat flour" or "enriched wheat flour" fool you. During processing, the two most nutritious parts of the wheat, the bran and the germ, are removed. During the processing from wheat to white flour, many of the nutrients are pulled out of the product. "Wheat flour" or "enriched wheat flour" is essentially the same as white flour, unless the label explicitly lists "*whole* wheat flour." Whole wheat flour is a healthier alternative. Examples of white flour products that contribute to weight gain include white bread, white pasta, white pizza dough, flour tortillas, biscuits, bread, crackers, crepes, croutons, dumplings, pancakes, piecrust, pretzels, waffles, and noodles.

Furthermore, white flour is bleached nearly the same

way you bleach your clothing. When you eat white flour, you're eating some of those bleaching agents, which increases the toxic overload in the body.

Sodas and Sports Drinks

It's possible to consume more calories from sodas and other sweet drinks than from any other single food; there are about 250 calories in one 20-ounce bottle of soda. Sodas are empty calories because they do not provide nutrients. If you are a heavy soda drinker, simply replacing your soda intake with water is a good way to lose a considerable amount of weight within a year. Diet sodas are lower in calories and are a better choice if you are trying to lose weight, even though they have hidden side effects due to the artificial sweeteners used in them. In the previous chapter, I discussed healthier beverage options.

Processed Meats

Foods like hot dogs, salami, pepperoni, bacon, many sausages, etc., are poor-quality meats and are often full of nitrates and other preservatives that are bad for your digestion and health. It's possible to find healthier varieties of these foods in stores like Whole Foods or at butcher shops that do not contain nitrates or preservatives. If you do need to splurge once in a while by having bacon or sausage, find these less-processed, healthier varieties.

Cow's Milk Products

Milk that you think does the body good may actually be contributing to the deterioration of your bones and organs. Cow's milk is too difficult for the human body to break down, which means it will leave waste residue in the body that piles up over time if consumed on a regular basis. Just as breast milk is designed for human infants, cow's milk is designed for baby cows, not for us. Additionally, because the milk is pasteurized, most of its positive attributes, like its enzymes, are cooked out. It is true that dairy products contain calcium, but they also contain animal proteins that are very difficult for the body to digest. And calcium can be obtained from other food sources, such as nuts, seeds, and green leafy veggies like kale, spinach, and dandelion greens, which are high in absorbable calcium and also provide many other essential nutrients.

Another problem with cow's milk is that the cows are injected with growth hormones and antibiotics to help them produce milk, and we take those hormones and antibiotics directly into our bloodstream when we consume milk products. Because milk is considered a high mucus-forming food, it leads to allergies, infections, colds, and asthma—ailments many kids experience because they consume more milk products than adults do. Children end up with mucus buildup very early in their life.

Dairy products made from the milk of goats and sheep are better than those made from cow's milk, particularly if they are raw. There are also non-dairy milk options, such as almond, rice, hemp, or soy milk (unsweetened). The natural enzymes in goat's milk are far closer to those in humans, so we're able to digest goat's milk significantly better. If you love cheese, consider switching to goat cheese, particularly in its raw, unpasteurized form, which can be a good treat for you. Sheep's milk cheese is the next best choice.

If you still decide to consume products made with cow's milk, buy organic and no-fat or low-fat brands because they are more nutritious.

Diet Foods That Make You Fat

There are many products marketed as "diet" because they have some reduced amount of sugar or fat. But without looking at all the ingredients, you won't be able to identify the hidden ones that may contribute to weight gain. Also, there are many low-calorie products that have little to no nutritional value and provide very little health benefit.

Diet Sodas

Although diet sodas are better than regular sodas because they have no sugar, diet sodas still cause some health and weight issues. The artificial sweeteners in diet sodas are thought to potentially cause some health problems, including cancer. Have you ever wondered why people walk around all day drinking diet sodas but they are not thin? Diet sodas are made from chemicals and have no nutritional value. When the body finds nothing recognizable as nutrition, the brain sends signals to be fed something nutritional, which creates cravings for more. Diet sodas make you crave fattening foods. If you are addicted to sodas and diet sodas, you could drink green tea, which is a fat burner and helps you lose more weight, while still getting your caffeine fix for the day. You could also try plain water. If plain water does not sound appealing, try adding a bit of lemon or cranberry juice to it. However, don't replace soda with a lot of store-bought juices, because they contain a lot of sugar and additives that cause weight gain.

Sugar-Free Baked Goods

You have to be careful that sugar-free baked goods don't have the same amount of or more fat than the original recipes. Although the serving size may say 0 grams of sugar, it could very well have 9 grams of fat, which can also cause weight gain. Until you totally wean yourself off sugar and sweets, to satisfy your sweet tooth, try graham crackers, which have less sugar (about a teaspoon less per serving than most other cookies) and very little fat, about 2 grams per serving. They provide a subtle sweetness without the tremendous number of calories contained in cakes and cookies.

Fat-Free Dressings

Trying to avoid fats altogether should not be the goal. There are healthy fats that are very good for the body. Most fat-free products are generally higher in sugar, which defeats the overall purpose of eating a fat-free product to lose weight. Try an oil-based, reduced-fat dressing that contains olive or canola oil (healthy fats) and has 2 to 4 grams of fat per serving.

High-Protein Diet Bars (Power Bars) and Shakes

When the body receives a protein or power bar, it tries to break down the sugar and chemicals in it, but when these elements cannot be fully digested by the body, the excess ends up being stored in the body as fat. A better alternative is an avocado, which is high in protein, and because it is in its natural state, the body knows how to break it down completely and use it to fuel the body. (See Chapter 11 for a list of other healthy, high-protein snacks.)

Fruit Snacks

Fruit snacks have added sugars and artificial ingredients that counteract any potential nutritional benefits they might have. Don't get fooled by marketing if the package says the product is made with real fruit or fruit juices. Instead, read the list of ingredients on the nutrition label; if the product has a high number of grams of sugar, it is fattening. A better alternative is to eat fresh fruit. Just get the real thing and gain all the benefits of fruits. Unlike fruit snacks, real fruit is rich in fiber, phytonutrients, and cancer-fighting antioxidants. You should even watch out for dried fruit because it usually contains a lot of added sugar as well.

Artificial Sweeteners

You know them in those little yellow, pink, and blue packages that are generally marketed as "sugar substitutes." Most people don't realize that even though artificial sweeteners generally have zero calories, they can still contribute to weight gain. These artificial sweeteners increase appetite by sending false signals to the brain that sweet food is on the way. The brain subsequently becomes confused when sweet food never arrives and so it never gives the signal that you are satisfied. You develop a sweet tooth and sugar cravings throughout the day, sometimes causing you to eat more sugar.

Let's look at aspartame, in particular. Despite its zero calories, studies have shown that aspartame can, in fact, induce weight gain. Some researchers believe that the two main ingredients in aspartame, phenylalanine and aspartic acid, stimulate the release of insulin and leptin, hormones that instruct our bodies to store fat, according to a study called "Physiological Mechanisms Mediating Aspartame-Induced Satiety."

The best choice for a calorie-free sweetener is stevia, an herb that grows naturally in parts of Paraguay and Brazil and is now widely available in this country. You don't need much of it—according to studies, it's thirty times sweeter than sugar. Yet it does not raise blood sugar levels or cause rapid-onset cravings the way simple sugars do. A study published in the *Journal of Ethno-Pharmacology* found that stevia dilates the blood vessels and helps to prevent high blood pressure. It also helps to regulate the digestive system, encourages the growth of friendly bacteria, and helps us detoxify the body and excrete more urine naturally.

Just because a product is labeled low-fat or fat free doesn't always mean the product is not still high in sugar, salt, and calories. You should get in the habit of reading food labels to ensure the product is healthy and nutritional. However, if you limit or avoid the food items listed above, you will have a much easier time getting to your ideal weight.

PART 3

The DEM System for Burning Fat, Losing Weight, and Getting Healthy

The DEM System for Burning Fat, Losing Weight, and Getting Healthy

The DEM System addresses the underlying causes of weight gain, which are:

- Toxic overload
- Hormonal imbalances
- Sluggish metabolism
- Unhealthy eating habits

The DEM System provides a quick-start plan for dramatically but naturally addressing all of the above factors in your efforts to lose weight and improve your health. You should look forward to an exciting journey. The DEM System is not a temporary solution to weight loss. Expect your life to change for the better because you will not only lose weight, have more energy, and look better, you will likely, for the first time ever, desire healthy, nutrient-rich foods.

The DEM System will provide your body with foods, supplements, and detox methods that help the body get rid of toxins, correct hormonal imbalances, and crave healthy foods. Your body does the rest automatically. It has a natural ability to heal and restore balance; the body can renew and rejuvenate itself naturally. Your body's natural intelligence does know what to do if you simply get out of the way. If you give it a rest and a chance to repair and heal, it will. Also, by eliminating the major sources of foods that cause toxins and disease, such as sugar and flour products, bad fats/oils, and food allergens, your body can heal itself.

The DEM System focuses on good nutrition and healthy eating. You will learn what to eat and how to make your body burn fat more efficiently while controlling cravings and hunger. You will learn which foods actually boost your metabolism and target excess fat in the body. The focus of the DEM System revolves around "superfoods" that detoxify and cleanse the body of fat while also providing the highest sources of protein, carbs, and fiber that help the pounds melt away.

Following the DEM System will provide you with the following benefits:

- You will flush away waste and excess fat quickly and learn how to keep your body fat-resistant for years to come.

- You will remove years from your face, as fine lines and wrinkles diminish, allowing you to experience a "second youth."

- You will experience weight loss due to the elimination of excess waste. Impacted fecal matter in your colon and digestive system cause excess weight in the body.

- You will have more energy as your body responds better to healthy foods. By removing excess waste, your body will absorb even more nutrients from the foods you eat, leaving you feeling energized and well.

- You will see a decrease in feelings of indigestion, bloating, and fatigue after eating.

- You will learn new ways to make time for sleep, rest, and relaxation and simple, easy ways to get moving and speed up your metabolism without going to a gym.

- You will get rid of unhealthy cravings. By changing your eating habits for just one month, you will become aware of how different foods affect you, allowing you to begin avoiding foods that are bad for you.

- You will feel more balanced and happy due to a healthy balance among your body's hormonal signals.

What you won't get on the DEM System are the following:

- *Calorie counting.* There will be no calorie counting or measuring grams of food.

- *Exercise regimen.* You won't have to exercise in the gym for hours a week (unless you choose to do so for the other health benefits exercise provides).

- *Going hungry.* You shouldn't experience severe hunger during this program if you follow my recommendations.

- *Cravings.* Although you may experience cravings during the first phase, you shouldn't expect them after that. It is necessary to break the addiction to many unhealthy foods that you've been eating for so long.

- *Bland, boring foods.* You also don't have to worry about disgusting or tasteless food. The food choices are delicious with plenty of options to choose from.

- *Slow results.* People often complain that it takes too long to see the benefits and get results from traditional diets, but you can expect rapid weight loss on the DEM System.

Ready-Set-Go: Preparing to Begin the DEM System

Whenever I'm planning a long vacation or trip, I take time to find a nice hotel, get a flight, and pick out the clothes I want to wear. In other words, I take time to get ready. The same is true for the journey toward health and wellness on which you are about to embark. Take time to properly prepare for the program. It will make your transition easier, and you will be more likely to succeed in following the program.

Spend several days preparing to begin the DEM System. Gather the foods, supplies, supplements, and any additional resources (e.g., books). You may even want to cut back on foods that will be eliminated during the detox phase, such as caffeine, sugar, sodas, processed or packaged junk and fast foods, and white-flour products, a few days before you begin. Eliminating items from your diet in a systematic way will help minimize potential withdrawal symptoms and jumpstart the process to weight loss and optimal health.

An Overview of the Three Key Elements of the DEM System

DEM stands for Detox, Eat, and Move. The system focuses on helping you detoxify, cleanse, and reset your taste buds so that you desire healthy, natural foods. Each of the three key elements of the program includes detoxification methods, food and beverage choices, and supplements to enhance your progress.

D Is for DETOX. Get rid of toxins in the body for fast

weight loss. You will detoxify the body through elimination of certain foods for three weeks, as well as use other detoxification methods that eliminate toxic waste from your body. As you do this, you will get rid of unhealthy foods and reprogram your taste buds to desire healthy, nutrient-rich foods.

E Is for EAT. Eat "clean and balanced" foods for permanent weight loss. You will learn the method of eating clean and balanced foods to help you achieve your ideal weight. You will enjoy the healthy, whole-food eating plan you started in the detoxification phase but will begin to reintroduce some of the foods you avoided and determine which ones will have negative consequences on your health or weight-loss efforts. When reintroducing them, you can monitor their effects on your health. As an example, if you drink milk and find that you get a stuffy nose, it is best that you stay away from milk because it is creating intolerances in your system.

M Is for MOVE. Get moving without going to the gym or "working out." You can begin this part of the program right away. I will help you incorporate easy and effective ways of getting physically active, as well as strengthening your muscles, into your everyday life.

I've designed this three-phase system with not only your body in mind but also your overall health and well-being. You will get rid of excess fat in your body and reverse some of your health issues and ailments, restoring your body to optimal health. Now that it has become easier and more economical to get access to better-quality organic foods and supplements, optimal health is achievable for everyone. We can find most of what we need right in our grocery store.

There are many large and small changes that you can make in your lifestyle and diet that have an immediate impact and enormous improvement on your health. However you go about doing the DEM System, the journey will be uniquely yours, and the changes you experience will be perfect and appropriate for you.

CHAPTER TEN

DETOX (D) — Get Rid of Toxins for Fast Weight Loss

The DEM System is geared for weight loss as well as detoxification. You will get the benefits of weight loss, but more importantly, you will transition to living a healthier, more vibrant life. This detox phase is designed to transition you to eating whole, unprocessed, natural foods as well as removing the most common unhealthy food choices. During this phase, you are reeducating your body and programming your taste buds to enjoy foods that help you lose weight and keep it off. You will also eliminate foods to which you may have sensitivities that cause inflammation in the body. It is not uncommon to lose up to fifteen pounds in this three-week phase. Besides weight loss, you can expect to feel more energetic, to sleep better, and to be rid of chronic sinus and digestive problems and recurring headaches.

In this phase, which lasts for three weeks, you will begin the cleansing process by focusing on foods that cleanse and detoxify the body, while avoiding foods that cause weight gain, excess toxins, and inflammation in the body. You will reprogram your taste buds to crave whole, natural, healthy foods as opposed to high-sugar junk foods. You will begin to enjoy a new variety of foods while still losing weight during this three-week period. During this phase, you will be eliminating the Big 6, the most addictive, unhealthy, and fattening foods. At the end of the three weeks, when you can begin to reintroduce these foods, you will likely have lost your taste for them. Once your body doesn't crave them, you will have a balanced body chemistry that lets you eat them in moderation, from time to time, but not every day.

You will be reprogramming your body to enjoy and crave natural and healthy foods that limit insulin production in the body, which is an underlying cause of excess fat in the body. You will also eat foods that build and maintain muscle tone with very little effort. In choosing what to eat, you will balance carbohydrates, proteins, and fats at every meal. You will not be counting calories: the focus is on quality of calories, not quantity. Consuming large amounts of fresh vegetables, fruits, grains, beans, nuts, seeds, and fats will rebuild your cells following detox. If you love to eat like I do, you will be glad to know that for the three weeks of this phase, you will enjoy eating delicious, nutrient-rich foods and you won't be hungry. Don't worry about failing or giving up if discipline is not your strong suit. Here's what you do. If you slip up or eat some of the foods you're supposed to avoid, just continue to avoid the Big 6 foods and keep pressing forward. Challenge yourself to stick to the program, but don't beat yourself up too badly if you slip up. If you find that one or two items, like coffee, is too difficult to give up, just avoid everything but caffeine and make the most of the program anyway. That is still better than giving up entirely. Maybe the next time you try it, you'll be ready to give up all of the Big 6 foods. It's all about making good progress, not being perfect! Another option is to find a friend, co-worker, or family member to follow the DEM System with so you can support and encourage one another. This is your journey. Make it your own, enjoy it, and make it appropriate for you.

Big 6 Foods to Avoid
During This Phase

In this phase, you will avoid the following Big 6 foods and beverages for three weeks. The Big 6 foods to avoid are either fattening, addictive, and/or unhealthy. The Big 6 foods to avoid are:

1. Caffeine drinks (tea, coffee, soda, diet soda)
2. Sugar (candy, sweets, cookies, cakes, processed foods that contain sugar)
3. White Carbs (white bread, white rice, white pasta, white potatoes)
4. Meats (fish, chicken, beef)
5. Dairy (eggs, milk, cheese)
6. Alcohol (liquor, beer, wine)

In this phase, I recommend that you abstain from the Big 6 for three weeks and replace them with healthy, whole, plant-based foods, such as nutritious vegetables, whole grains, beans, fruits, and nuts.

When people decide to refrain from eating the Big 6, the first thing they ask me is, "What in the world is left to eat?" But you'll discover a whole array of delicious, natural foods that make you feel healthy and energetic. You won't have to starve or feel hungry because you will be eating—

just different foods than your body is used to eating. As in the entire DEM System, you will not be counting calories or measuring carbs, proteins, or fats, just learning to enjoy healthier foods that will fuel your body. Also, if you are satisfied with the food choices and your weight loss during this phase, you can continue in it as long as you like as it has very healthy, natural food choices. However, for those who want to begin to add some of the Big 6 foods back into their diet, progressing to the next phase will guide you toward a long-term, healthy eating plan.

Foods to Eat During This Phase

To ensure you get the highest-quality foods, you may have to visit a local health food store, not just a regular grocery store. A local health food store will have more natural, organic foods with more options as well. I personally never thought I would crave raw seeds and nuts, but I just love them for an afternoon snack, particularly sunflower seeds and cashews. They sure beat the candy I'd eat after raiding the vending machine most afternoons before I began the DEM System.

Breakfast Foods

- *Whole-grain or mixed-grain cereals.* There are a variety of hot and cold cereals that contain whole grain or mixed grain. Oatmeal is a great choice, and you can use stevia or fresh fruit to sweeten to taste. My favorite two brands, with a large variety of whole-grain cereals, is Bob's Red Mill products or Ezekial 4:9.

Lunch/Dinner Foods

- *Vegetables.* A few good choices include spinach, kale,

collard greens, broccoli, cauliflower, green beans, asparagus, Brussels sprouts, zucchini, eggplant, squash, tomatoes, and mushrooms.

- *Whole grains.* Brown or wild rice, whole grain crackers, buckwheat, quinoa. Two of my favorite brands of whole grain food products is by Ezekiel 4:9, found at www.foodforlife.com and Bob's Red Mill products.

- *Salads.* Make yourself luxurious salads using mixed greens, romaine lettuce, spinach, arugula, carrots, mushrooms, cucumber, radicchio, endive, peppers, avocado, tomato, and radishes.

- *Beans and legumes.* Though they are considered starches, beans and legumes are especially healthy kinds because they are high in fiber and low in fat. Go wild eating black beans, lima beans, kidney beans, fava beans, butter beans, lentils, chickpeas, and black-eyed peas. Canned beans are fine, but you may want to rinse some of the salt off them before cooking.

- *Tofu, tempeh, and faux meats.* Sauté, bake, or grill tofu and tempeh, and mix them with vegetables and brown rice. There are also good vegetarian meat substitutes for burgers, sausage, or chicken patties available.

Snacks

- *Fruits.* A few good choices include apples, blackberries, blueberries, raspberries, strawberries, cherries, peaches, goji berries, grapefruits, and oranges.

- *Nuts and seeds.* These include almonds, walnuts, macadamia nuts, cashews, soy nuts, sunflower seeds, pumpkin seeds, sesame seeds, hemp seeds, and freshly ground flaxseeds, just to name a few. Buy organic raw nuts and seeds, when possible.

- *Other snack choices*. Rice cakes, flax crackers, unsweetened peanut butter, and popcorn (lightly seasoned with sea salt is fine).

Cooking Ingredients

- *Cooking oils*. The best choices are extra-virgin olive oil, organic canola, sunflower and safflower oils, and walnut oil.

- *Seasonings*. Use Celtic Sea salt, garlic, onions, ginger, and tamari. Do not use regular table salt.

- *Oils* to use on salads. The best choices are flaxseed oil, avocado oil, and olive oil.

- *Gluten-free flours*. Good choices are flours that contain rice, beans, oats, whole wheat, buckwheat, soy, barley, potato, cornmeal, flaxseed, nuts, seeds, quinoa, or tapioca.

- *Non-dairy butters*. Use nut or seed butters, such as almond butter, or vegan butter. Be sure the butters are unsweetened.

- *Sweeteners*. Stevia is especially good for cereals, smoothies, and baked goods. Agave nectar is another option to use in moderation.

Beverages

In Chapter 8, I discussed some of the best beverage options and explained the specific health benefits they provide. The recommended beverages to drink during this phase are listed below:

- Water

- Coconut water

- Fresh-squeezed juices

- Herbal caffeine-free teas like mint or chamomile

- Non-dairy milk, such as unsweetened almond, rice, hemp, or soy milk

Detoxification Methods
That Support This Phase

Detoxifying the body and eliminating toxins can be accomplished through various detoxification methods, as discussed in Chapter 5. During this three-week detoxification phase, I consider it mandatory that you take colon-cleansing and liver cleansing herbs/supplements. You need to rapidly eliminate toxins from your body to avoid feeling sick and to minimize detox symptoms. All the other detox methods listed are optional, but I would strongly encourage you to pick two or three of the others on a long-term basis, as you have the time and money to do so.

Some people notice a change for the better in their health and energy levels within a few days; however, for others, it may take a few months. Everyone's toxic overload is different, and many factors come into play, such as your health status, weight, metabolism, age, and genetics. So be patient and steadfast through the detoxification process.

Supplements to Take
During This Phase

In Chapter 8, I provide a list of supplements that will help you control your weight, achieve optimal health, fight disease, and slow the aging process. At a minimum, you should include the green drink and fiber during this phase as they are critical for detoxification. You can look to include other supplements from chapter 8 after the 21-day detox phase.

What to Expect
During This Phase

You may be surprised at how good you feel after this phase—lighter and more energetic. You may experience greater mental clarity. Many people who thought being sluggish and lethargic was a normal way of living are pleasantly surprised at how great they feel.

As a result of this detox phase, you will have given your body a chance to break free from cravings and addictive eating habits. You may have some cravings, and there may be some days when the process will seem difficult, but you will begin to see the light at the end of the tunnel. Some individuals don't experience any cravings at all.

Expect and Welcome Detox Symptoms

You may experience some detoxification symptoms, and their severity will depend on how toxic you were to begin with. You should expect and welcome detox symptoms because, although they can be unpleasant, they are a sign of progress. Your body is addicted to the Big 6 foods, and as you break those addictions, you will be learning for the first time how dependent your body has become on those foods.

Typical detox symptoms include the following:

- *Cravings.* As your body detoxifies, it craves foods it was used to eating, such as meat, dairy, sugar, and caffeine. Cravings may last for several hours or several days, but they will begin to decrease as your body gets rid of its toxic overload.

- *Headaches, pains, nausea.* If you drink a lot of coffee, expect headaches during the first few days. You may also experience physical aches and joint pains or even nausea.

- *Fatigue.* Allow time to rest during this detoxification phase, as eliminating toxins will drain you and make you feel exhausted. Just take it easy and rest.

- *Skin rashes.* Skin rashes, or even acne, are signs that your body is excreting toxins through your skin, which is the body's largest organ of elimination. By doing the colonics or taking the colon-cleansing herbs, you can minimize the rashes and breakouts.

- *Irritability.* Not eating some of your favorite foods will make you feel irritable and bored, so expect to be a little cranky. This is a good time to avoid social events as well.

Summary of the Detoxification Phase (Phase 1)

Here's a quick recap of what you need to do during this 21-day detoxification phase for rapid weight loss and renewed health and energy. Many people end up staying in this phase for six to eight weeks because they love the rapid weight loss, increased energy, improved digestion, and clearer skin. Feel free to do so as well.

- *Avoid the Big 6 foods.* The Big 6 foods that need to be avoided during this phase to detoxify the body are provided in this chapter. Food and beverage choices to eat and drink during this phase are also provided.

- *Complete a Colon Cleanse and a Liver Cleanse.* You should use both colon cleansing and liver cleansing herbs/supplements during the 21-day detoxification phase. For the colon cleanse, recommended products to choose from include Mag07 by Aerobic Life, Dr. Natura's Colonix, or Blessed Herbs Colon-cleansing kit. For a liver cleanse, recommended products to choose from include Liver Rescue by Healthforce and Livatone Plus by Dr. Sandra Cabot. Feel free to select one or two other detox methods, as described in Chapter 5; these other detox methods are optional during this phase.

- *Drink a Green Drink and Take a Fiber Supplement Every Morning.* The green drink and fiber are mandatory during the 21-day detox phase and will go far to help you detoxify and cleanse the body. Recommended products for the green drink are Green Vibrance or Vitamineral Green. For a fiber supplement, I like Sprinkle Fiber by Fiber35 because you can just add a scoop right into your green drink every morning. After the 21-day detox phase, you can look to include additional supplements that are described in Chapter 8.

In Conclusion

The body is fully capable of healing, rejuvenating, and restoring itself to optimum health, and detoxification allows you to do just that. The twenty-one days should give your body sufficient time to reprogram your taste buds, and you will begin to enjoy healthier, more natural foods, permanently changing your unhealthy eating habits.

After the twenty-one days of this detoxification phase, you will experience great health benefits. You will begin to naturally slim down. You will begin to think more clearly. You will feel energized and more alive. You will notice a clearer complexion. You will feel happier and balanced. And, most important, detoxifying the body on a long-term basis will ensure your body doesn't accumulate toxic waste that leads to excess fat in the body.

CHAPTER ELEVEN

EAT (E) — Eat Clean and Balanced Foods for Permanent Weight Loss

In earlier chapters, we discussed which foods are healthy and contribute to weight gain and which ones contribute to weight loss. In this chapter, we focus on how much to eat, what types of food, and what combinations of foods are best for the body.

You will enjoy the healthy, whole-food eating plan you started in the detoxification phase but will begin to reintroduce some of the foods you avoided and determine which ones will have negative consequences on your health or weight-loss efforts. When reintroducing them, you can monitor their effects on your health. As you begin to reintroduce certain foods, you will need to observe how they affect your weight and how you feel. If certain foods still cause you to have allergic reactions (bloating, gas, headaches) and hinder your weight-loss goals, you will want to continue to avoid them. You may want to keep a journal at this time to keep track of what you eat every day and the feelings or allergic symptoms associated with certain foods.

The foods in the DEM System will help you balance

179

hormones, decrease hunger, regulate your metabolism, and remove toxins that lead to chronic disease. The foods in the DEM System, which include lean proteins, good carbs, and healthy fats at each meal, have the following characteristics:

- Low in sugar
- Primarily natural, whole, raw, or organic
- High in fiber and omega-3 fatty acids
- High in vitamins, minerals, and nutrients
- Low in sodium

Transitioning from the Detox Phase to the Eat Phase

Here are a few key guidelines to help you transition from the Detox Phase to the Eat Phase. This will help ensure that you continue to lose weight as you transition to the Eat Phase.

Regarding the Big 6 Foods that you avoided in Phase 1 (Detox Phase), here's how you should transition these foods back into your diet:

1. *Caffeine drinks:* Feel free to add a limited amount of caffeine back into your diet. Caffeine can speed up your metabolism by five to eight percent, which helps to burn about 100 to 175 calories a day. This does not mean you should overdo it and drink several cups of coffee per day, but having one cup of coffee will not have adverse effects on your weight-loss goals. Additionally, green tea, my favorite metabolism booster, is found to provide many health benefits to the body as well as help your body burn fat. Green tea is highly recommended as a daily drink.

2. *Sugar:* I explained that sugar is highly addictive and how it makes us fat and sick in Chapter 3; there is no good reason to bring sugar back into your diet. Of course, we are referring to white refined sugar, high-fructose corn syrup, etc. You should continue to use stevia and other natural sweeteners that don't have adverse effects on your health and weight-loss goals.

3. *White Carbs:* You will continue to avoid white carbs, such as white bread, white rice, white pasta, white flour, and white potatoes. Feel free to use healthier alternatives, such as whole-grain bread, brown or wild rice, whole-grain pasta, whole-wheat flours, and sweet potatoes.

4. *Meats:* Meats provide the body with lean proteins, which are extremely effective for helping to maintain muscle, burn calories, and balance blood sugar levels. So, during this phase, you want to transition meats (lean protein) back into your diet. A good approach is to bring back fish for the first week, then bring back chicken, and the following week, you can have lean red meat on occasion. Red meat contains a lot of saturated fat, so try to limit your intake to two or three times a week. Instead, eat more protein from fish, poultry, and vegetable sources, such as brown rice, beans, and nuts.

5. *Dairy:* If you discovered that you're allergic to dairy (cow's milk) during the Detox Phase, then you want to continue avoiding it. However, eggs, low-fat cheese, and non-dairy milk (such as almond milk or soy milk) are still great long-term dairy options.

6. *Alcohol:* If you were a drinker before the Detox Phase, you're probably anxious to bring alcohol back into your diet. However, you should still drink alcohol in moderation. Be mindful how harsh alcohol can be on the liver; you will want to do liver cleanses every few months if you consume a great deal of alcohol.

Detox Methods: In the Detox Phase, you completed a colon cleanse and a liver cleanse. For maintenance, you can do colon cleansing and liver cleansing as you feel your toxic overload building up in your system, and, for most, this is typically every three to six months. However, for those who maintain healthy eating, drink clean or alkaline water, or take little to no prescriptions or supplements, you may only need to do colon or liver cleansing once a year. This is a great time to revisit Chapter 5 and begin incorporating other detox methods into your routine.

Supplements: In the Detox Phase, the green drink and fiber were mandatory supplements. You can continue both of these supplements, as they will continue to help you improve your health, cleanse your digestive tract, and help you achieve your weight-loss goals. During this phase, you also want to consider adding any additional supplements that are described in Chapter 8. Keep in mind that these supplements are not required but can be added to address specific ailments and digestive issues.

One Final Note: You must understand the difference between "body fat" and "stubborn body fat." You can burn body fat by eating healthy "clean and balanced" meals and being physically active, but to lose stubborn body fat, you will have to correct hormonal imbalances, as discussed in Chapter 6. When eating healthy and being physically active are not enough to achieve your weight-loss goals, hormonal imbalances are the likely culprit. If you are challenged to lose weight or your weight loss stalls, you will have to incorporate methods to balance your hormones, as discussed in Chapter 6. Additionally, be sure you've include some of the metabolism boosters discussed in Chapter 7 to help your body burn more fat effortlessly.

What Are "Clean and Balanced" Foods?

As discussed earlier, "clean" foods are primarily natural, whole, raw, or organic—foods that the body can effectively digest and utilize for energy without leaving excess waste or toxins in the body. Clean foods include lean proteins, good carbs, and healthy fats. "Balanced" foods mean that you will balance your meals by eating protein every time you eat a carbohydrate. So, if you have carbohydrates, you want to always include protein. Maintaining this balance between proteins and carbs is a very simple but incredibly effective method for preventing insulin spikes and aiding the body in burning fat.

Why protein every time you eat? Protein counteracts the body's overreaction to carbohydrates, which cause insulin spikes and fat storage. Proteins will also help you feel full longer and thus will help prevent overeating and food cravings. Protein will also help you build and maintain muscle mass, and, as we've learned, muscle naturally burns more calories than fat.

Eating clean and balanced foods will help you lose weight for all of the following reasons.

- It will help you address the underlying reasons your body stores fat.
- You will learn which foods will help you stay thin and maintain your healthy weight.
- You will have more control over your insulin and blood sugar levels.
- You will burn fat, especially the belly fat and love handles.
- You will gain control of your appetite and cravings.

Twelve Principles for Eating "Clean and Balanced" Foods

Look at the principles below as your instructions on how to eat "clean and balanced" foods.

- *Principle #1: Choose nutrient-rich foods, not empty calories.* This means you will eat foods that are high in vitamins, minerals, phytonutrients, fiber, and omega-3 fatty acids. Eating junk foods is like eating empty calories. You want your calories to provide you with nutritional benefits that will help you heal your body and maintain a permanently healthy weight. Before you eat anything, ask yourself, is this a healthy, nutrient-rich food or empty calories? Commit to be mindful of everything you eat.

- *Principle #2: Eat protein with every meal.* Eat protein with every meal, and eat it first before the carbohydrates or fats. You can also eat protein by itself. Eating protein foods does not cause insulin spikes, making them an important staple of eating clean and balanced foods.

184

- *Principle #3: Always "balance" carbohydrates with protein.* Whenever you eat a carbohydrate, eat some protein along with it. As a general guideline, the protein should be about half the amount of the carbohydrates. For example, if you had 30 grams of carbohydrates, then eat about 15 grams of protein along with it to prevent insulin spikes that cause excess fat to be stored in the body. You can use food labels to determine how much carbs (or "net carbs") and protein is in food. (See the examples at the end of this section to better understand how to balance carbohydrates with protein at each meal.)

- *Principle #4: Don't overeat carbohydrates.* It is important to not overeat carbohydrates. Limit yourself to no more than two servings of high-carbohydrate foods at any one meal or snack. This will prevent excess carbohydrates from being stored as fat. If you are still hungry, then eat more vegetables to satisfy your hunger. Do not try to eat other high-carbohydrate foods, which will convert to fat in your body, or too much protein, which will hinder weight loss by adding extra calories. One serving of high-carbohydrate foods is about 1/2 cup or 15 grams of carbohydrates. So, the maximum amount of high-carb foods you should eat at any one meal is two servings, which is 30 grams or about 1 cup, *always balanced with a high-protein food.*

- *Principle #5: Avoid sugar, salt, and trans fat.* We discussed a number of foods that cause weight gain and are bad for your health. However, these three are at the top of the list. Try to avoid them at all costs. They have no nutritional value and are simply bad for your health. Chapter 3 is entirely devoted to explaining how detrimental sugar is. Salt is also bad for your health and causes bloating, swelling, and fluid retention. As far as trans fat, the good news is that the FDA regulates it, and food manufacturers now have to list how much trans fat is in each serving when trans fats exceed 0.5 grams per serving.

- *Principle #6: Eat at least five servings of fruits and veggies each day.* Fruit breaks down faster in the body than any other food, leaving us fueled and energized, and because it is a highly cleansing food, it leaves no toxic residue and acts as a strong cleanser for the body. You need to eat vegetables if you want to get thin, as studies have shown that those who eat a large variety of vegetables have the least amount of body fat. Veggies and fruits are naturally balanced because they contain both protein and carbohydrates. They are made up of mostly water and fiber, so they can be eaten in larger quantities. However, there are a few exceptions. Consumption of corn and potatoes should be minimal and, of course, always be balanced with protein.

- *Principle #7: Limit your intake of red meat to two to three times per week.* Red meat contains a lot of saturated fat, so try to limit your intake to two or three times a week. Instead, eat more protein from fish, poultry, and vegetable sources, such as brown rice, beans, and nuts, which contain good essential fats.

- *Principle #8: Eat two healthy snacks per day.* Snacks keep you from getting hungry between meals. Eating snacks allows you to feed your body every three to four hours, which keeps your metabolism revved up. See the list of healthy snacks provided later in this chapter.

- *Principle #9: Eat at least 30 grams of fiber per day.* Numerous studies have shown that high-fiber diets help you lose weight and protect against heart disease, stroke, and certain kinds of cancer. Chapter 8 provides a list of foods that are high in fiber as well as fiber supplements that help you to eat 30 grams of fiber per day.

- *Principle #10: Eat fruit by itself, one hour before or after meals.* The enzymes in fruit are digested better if the fruit is eaten alone. Therefore, fruit is a perfect snack food.

- *Principle #11: Eat four to five times a day.* You will lose weight more quickly if you eat four or five times a day as opposed to only three meals (or fewer). Try to eat every three to four hours, and think in terms of three meals and two healthy snacks. Each time you eat, you stimulate your metabolism for a short period of time; thus, the more often you eat, the more you speed up your metabolism. Eating every two to three hours feeds your muscles and starves fat.

- *Principle #12: Buy organic as much as possible.* Buy organic foods, which don't have chemical preservatives, food additives, hormones, pesticides, and antibiotics. Fresh organic foods are far less toxic than highly processed and packaged/frozen foods and leave less residue and waste in the body.

Here are some examples of how to "balance" carbohydrates with proteins (the protein food is listed in italics):

- Breakfasts
  - ✦ Oatmeal cooked in *fat-free* or *low-fat milk* (add fresh fruit to sweeten)
  - ✦ *Omelet* with *lean turkey sausage* and hash browns
  - ✦ An *egg* or *egg whites* with whole wheat toast
  - ✦ Pancakes or waffles with *lean pork sausage*
  - ✦ Unsweetened *yogurt* with whole grain cereal

- Lunch
  - ✦ *Tuna* on whole wheat bread with a garden salad
  - ✦ Low-fat, nitrate-free *lunch meat* on whole wheat bread
  - ✦ *Chili*, *bean*, or *pea soup* with whole-grain crackers
  - ✦ *Chicken* or *steak* in a Caesar salad
  - ✦ Grilled *chicken* sandwich on whole wheat bun
  - ✦ Grilled *salmon* with a garden salad

- Dinner
  - ✦ Lean *steak* with sweet potatoes and veggies
  - ✦ Grilled *salmon* with quinoa and veggies
  - ✦ Baked *chicken* with mashed potatoes and sautéed veggies
  - ✦ *Chicken* stir-fry with brown rice
  - ✦ Lean *sirloin steak* with *lima beans*
  - ✦ *Meatballs* with reduced-fat cheese on whole wheat pasta with salad

    ✦ *Chili* with whole-grain crackers and salad

- Snacks

    ✦ Unsweetened *peanut butter* with celery sticks

    ✦ Reduced-fat *cheese sticks* with an apple

    ✦ Unsweetened *yogurt* with fresh fruit

    ✦ Two tablespoons of *nuts* (almonds, macadamia, Brazil nuts) with fresh juice

    ✦ Carrot or celery sticks with a low-fat *cheese* spread

    ✦ Graham crackers with *low-fat* or *fat-free milk*

    ✦ Reduced fat *cheese sticks (string cheese)* with crackers

"Clean and Balanced" Food Choices

During this phase, you will eat clean and balanced foods from the lean proteins, good carbs, and healthy fats lists below. This section provides specific lists of some food choices for each category. This list is meant to give you many food choice options, but it does not represent the only foods that are suitable on the DEM System. Always use the principles above to select the right balance of lean proteins, good carbs, and healthy fats each day. The end result will provide the best balance of carbs, proteins, and fats to ensure that the rate at which your body breaks down your food into energy lends itself to meeting your weight-loss goals.

The following are daily guidelines for how much of each type of food to eat for a well-balanced diet.

- *Lean proteins* (30 percent of daily diet): Two or three servings (3 to 4 ounces per serving) of lean proteins, such as lean red meat, poultry, and fish

- *Good carbs* (45 percent of daily diet): At least five servings of fruits and vegetables/legumes (beans) and two or three servings of whole grains (1/2 cup = one serving)

- *Healthy fats* (25 percent of daily diet): One to two servings (about 1 ounce) of nuts and seeds per day and one to three tablespoons of healthy oils

LEAN PROTEINS		
Eat 2 or 3 servings (3 to 4 ounces per serving) of lean protein daily.		
Fish & Shellfish	Chicken & Turkey	Lean Red Meat
bass, calamari, catfish, clams, cod, crabmeat, flounder, grouper, haddock, halibut, lobster, mackerel, oysters, perch, wild salmon, sardines, scallops, shrimp, red snapper, sole, tilapia, trout, tuna	skinless chicken breasts, skinless Cornish hen, skinless turkey breast	lean beef, flank steak, sirloin, top round, London broil, pork tenderloin, pork rib chops, pork roast
	Dairy Products	
	eggs, protein drink/powder, goat and sheep's milk products, unsweetened yogurt, non-dairy milk such as unsweetened almond, rice, hemp, soy milk	

GOOD CARBS

Fruits: 2 servings or 2 whole fruits daily
Veggies/legumes: 3 to 4 cups daily
Whole grains: 2 to 3 three servings daily (1/2 cup = one serving)

Fruits	Veggies/Legumes	Whole Grains
apples, apricots, avocado, bananas, blackberries, blueberries, cantaloupe, cherries, cranberries, dates, figs, grapes, kiwi, grapefruit, guava, honeydew, lemon, lime, mango, nectarines, oranges, papaya, peaches, pears, pineapple, plums, pomegranate, prunes, raspberries, strawberries, tangerines, watermelon	alfalfa, artichokes, asparagus, beets and beet greens, broccoli, Brussels sprouts, cabbage, carrots, cauliflower, celery, chiles, cilantro, collard greens, cucumbers, dandelion greens, eggplant, fennel, garlic, green beans, kale, kelp, leeks, lettuce, mushrooms, mustard greens, okra, onion, parsley, parsnips, pea pods, peas, peppers, pumpkin, radishes, rhubarb, rutabaga, scallions, spinach, summer squash, sweet potato, tomato, turnips, turnip greens, watercress, yams, zucchini,	oatmeal, barley, bran, brown rice, buckwheat, bulgur wheat, cornmeal, millet, oats, oat bran, quinoa, rye, spelt, wheat germ, wild rice, whole-grain/gluten-free breads, whole-grain/gluten-free pastas, whole-grain cereals
	black beans, lentils, kidney beans, pinto beans, split peas, chickpeas (garbanzo beans), lima beans, butter beans, wax beans.	

HEALTHY FATS		
Nuts and Seeds: 1 or 2 servings (about 1 ounce) of nuts/seeds daily Healthy oils: 1 to 3 tablespoons daily		
Nuts	Seeds	Healthy Oils
almonds, Brazil nuts, cashews, chestnuts, coconut, hazelnuts, pecans, walnuts, macadamia nuts, pistachios	pumpkin seeds, sesame seeds, sunflower seeds, ground flaxseeds	avocado oil, canola oil, coconut oil, extra-virgin olive oil, flaxseed oil, fish oil, sesame oil, walnut oil

HEALTHY SNACKS		
Eat 2 healthy snacks per day.		
Healthy Low-Calorie Fruits and Veggies *(less than 100 calories)*	Healthy Low-Calorie Nuts and Seeds (Raw or Dry Roasted) *(less than 100 calories)*	Healthy High Protein/Low-Fat Snacks
• 1 large apple • 1/2 cup of unsweetened applesauce • 1 large orange • 1 medium grapefruit • 1 medium pear • 1 medium banana • 1 cup blueberries • 1 cup blackberries • 1 cup of raspberries • 1 cup of fresh cherries • 1 large nectarine • 2 medium peaches • 2 cups of grapes • 2 kiwis • 1 cup of celery/ celery sticks • 1/2 cup of baby carrots • 1 cup of broccoli • 1 cup of cauliflower	• 12 raw almonds • 8 walnut halves • 4 Brazil nuts • 1/2 oz. pumpkin seeds • 2 tablespoons sunflower seeds • 20 macadamia nuts • 20 peanuts	• 1 hard-boiled egg • 2 oz. tuna, lightly salted • low-fat cottage cheese, 1/2 cup • 1 oz. string goat cheese • 1 cup plain fat-free yogurt • 8 baked tortilla chips with 3 tablespoons salsa • 5 cups plain popcorn

Beverages to Drink
During This Phase

The beverages allowed during this phase include water, green tea, fresh-squeezed juices, coconut water, non-dairy milk options, an occasional diet soda if desired, and possibly a cup of coffee a day.

During periods of intense detoxification (like in Phase 1), I have abstained from drinking coffee, but at other times, I do enjoy drinking a cup a day. There are different schools of thought on whether coffee is bad for our health. Although coffee is acid forming, it is not too harsh on the liver; therefore, in my opinion, it will not interfere with your detoxification and cleansing steps for the long term. However, in the first phase of the DEM System, coffee should be avoided altogether. Eventually, you may find you desire less. In any case, coffee is not the biggest problem with staying slim and healthy. If you have a moderate amount of caffeine (about two cups of coffee or tea per day) and can sleep well at night and maintain energy and balance throughout the day, then caffeine may actually improve your health and metabolic fitness. I also recommend drinking green tea instead of coffee because it offers so many other health benefits. But if one (just one) cup of coffee (regular or decaf) in the morning is your guilty pleasure, then that should not pose a problem to your health.

Detox Methods and Supplements
That Support This Phase

All of the mandatory detox methods and supplements should be continued during this phase. You will want to continue trying different detox methods to identify those that are most effective for you. Additionally, you will want to consider taking nutritional supplements based upon your specific health concerns and issues. As an example, if you struggle with constipation or bloating, in addition to the green drink and fiber, probiotics and digestive enzymes would be good options to include during this phase.

Reintroducing Foods and Identifying Food Allergies

During this phase, you can begin introducing the foods that you were avoiding in Phase 1, but be aware of what is going on in your body during this time. During Phase 1 of the program, you may have eliminated foods you were unknowingly sensitive or even allergic to, and thus reintroducing these foods will trigger the symptoms those foods caused you to have.

Food allergies are not just the dramatic reactions that cause someone to end up in an emergency room with hives and shortness of breath from peanuts or something like that. That is an immediate and acute allergic reaction. It is not that common but can be very serious. However, there are reactions to foods that are much less dramatic but just as deadly. These are delayed allergies, and they are much more common, affecting millions of people. They are not easily diagnosed but they play a huge role in chronic illness and weight issues. About half of us have some foods that just don't agree with us and that cause a delayed allergic reaction. These delayed allergic reactions can cause symptoms anywhere from a few hours to several days after consumption. These delayed allergic reactions include weight gain, fluid retention, skin eruptions, fatigue, brain fog, irritable bowel syndrome, mood problems, headaches, sinus and nasal congestion, and muscle and joint pain or swelling. Eating foods you are allergic to causes inflammation, which ultimately leads to swelling and fluid retention. Getting rid of this fluid by reducing inflammation is a good thing and can happen with the detoxification methods described in this book. Your body can then start the healing process to allow you to achieve permanent weight loss and optimal health.

The foods most people are sensitive to are gluten, cow's milk, eggs, corn, peanuts, yeast, and wheat. Gluten is a special type of protein that is commonly found in rye, wheat, and barley and is responsible for the elastic texture of dough. It is found in most types of cereals and in many types of bread. Not all foods from the grain family contain gluten. Examples of grains that do not have gluten include wild rice, corn, buckwheat, millet, quinoa, oats, and soybeans. Because gluten is not a naturally occurring protein in the human body, studies have shown that it can cause general inflammation of the intestinal tract and can also damage the lining of the small intestine, making it difficult to absorb nutrients from foods.

Eliminating food allergies is the foundation for feeling better and dealing with chronic symptoms. To determine what foods you're allergic to, you can take a blood test for immunoglobulin G (IgG) antibodies to foods. This can be helpful but may not detect all food allergies. It may be more useful for you to identify food allergies by the process of elimination. This simply means you get rid of all potential foods that you think you may be allergic to for three or four weeks and then reintroduce them slowly, one at a time, and see how your system reacts to each one. Keep a food journal and take notes on how different foods affect how you feel or what symptoms they cause in your body. Write down what you eat, when you ate it, and how you felt for the next couple of days after you ate it. A journal will also record your overall weight loss and health and well-being.

For example, if you are trying to determine if you are allergic to wheat, you could eat a serving of Wheatena at breakfast and maybe a sandwich with wheat bread for lunch. Then observe your body carefully for the next two to three days. Watch to see if the wheat triggers any symptoms such as fluid retention, headaches, runny nose, or joint pain. If you experience such reactions or symptoms after you reintroduce the food, do not continue to include that food in your diet. Instead, wait and retry again in another month or two. If you still react negatively, you should just remove them from your diet altogether or visit a dietitian or nutritionist skilled in managing food allergies.

Because the foods we're most allergic or sensitive to are the ones we eat daily and crave, avoiding these foods can initially be a challenge. You should expect withdrawal symptoms and cravings for the addictive foods for only three to four days. Additionally, any of the allergic reactions could worsen during that timeframe. However, after those few days, you will feel better and begin to experience a sense of well-being. Symptoms such as brain fog, fluid retention, low energy, bloating, headaches, and other digestive complaints will lessen as well. Once you eliminate the offending foods, you allow your body to respond more efficiently to the rest of this program, and healing and weight loss can finally happen.

Enjoying Reward Meals in This Phase

Although maintaining weight loss is a life-long effort, we can still have some "reward meals" in this phase. The goal is to keep to your healthy new eating habits and have two "reward meals" on the weekends. I find that as much as I enjoy my reward meals, I begin to look forward to going back to my healthy eating habits because of how they make me look and feel. By adding these reward meals on the weekends, you keep your metabolism guessing. Since your metabolism is so well trained due to healthy eating habits, two reward meals on the weekend will not have an adverse affect on your weight-loss goals.

I would caution you that if you do eat a few reward meals and it causes you to revert back to your old eating habits, then avoid them altogether. It's not worth losing all the success and progress that you've gained. So give yourself permission to have less-than-healthy foods for two meals per week, with the understanding that you'll spend the rest of the week eating healthy, fat-burning, detoxifying foods that help keep you slim. For me, on the weekends—especially while I'm watching sports—I enjoy a thin crust pizza and a diet soda to the fullest.

Summary of the Eat "Clean and Balanced" Foods Phase (Phase 2)

Here's a quick recap of what you need to do during this phase for permanent weight loss and optimal health and vitality:

- *Follow the 12 Principles for Eating "Clean and Balanced" Foods.* These are your guidelines and instructions on how to ensure that what you eat helps you to lose body fat and control your weight long-term.

- *Select Your Food and Beverage Choices.* You were provided very specific food choices of lean proteins, good carbs, and healthy fats. Ensure that you get the proper balance of these foods daily. You should also watch for food allergies during this phase and continue to avoid any of the Big 6 items that make you feel sick or unhealthy. You can also enjoy reward meals if you are consistently following the "clean and balanced" food principles throughout the week.

- *Select Your Detox Methods and Nutritional Supplements.* All of the mandatory detox methods and supplements identified in Phase 1 should be continued during this phase. You will want to continue trying different detox methods and nutritional supplements to identify those that are most effective for you.

In Conclusion

During this phase, you will reach your desired weight and begin to enjoy optimal health. This phase teaches you everything you need to know for lifetime weight control. You can expect to experience not only a lean but also a healthy body, and a healthy body is a sexy body! You will begin to have fewer health issues and ailments and you will increase your vitality and well-being for life. You now understand which foods give your unique body the ability to stay slim, healthy, and energetic. You will continue to eat these foods and may even include a few "reward meals" on the weekend.

The dietary recommendations, food choices, and supplements in the DEM System can help your body stay clean and lean with no further toxic buildup to hinder your weight-loss efforts.

CHAPTER TWELVE

MOVE (M) — Get Moving Without Going to the Gym or "Working Out"

M ost of us spend the majority of the day sitting. We ride to work in a car, bus, or subway; we sit in front of an office computer working and then we ride back home only to watch our favorite television shows seated comfortably on the sofa. For many of us, the television has become our best friend and primary source of entertainment and babysitter for our children. Our bodies suffer because we sit for fourteen or fifteen hours or more a day. It weakens our heart, slows our metabolism, and weakens our muscle strength. We used to sit when we needed a break from our hectic day but now we sit over 80 percent of our waking hours.

The way we diet and exercise today does not work because it's unnatural. We can't just be sedentary for fifteen hours a day and think thirty minutes on the treadmill, only burning about 250 calories, is all the physical activity we need. We should be burning calories through constant physical activity throughout each day. Additionally, when we try to diet by selectively eliminating entire food groups, we often fail because we need all the foundation foods if our bodies are to stay healthy and lean. Our bodies thrive off nourishment and sustenance, not starvation and deprivation. A decade ago, there weren't half as many gyms as there are currently, and yet we didn't struggle with obesity the way we do today. A decade ago, people managed their weight because they moved; they moved to find food, they moved while they worked, and they moved for recreation. The modern electronic age has made us lazier than ever. At work, we don't even walk right down the hall to talk to a coworker. Instead, we use email or text messages. Our fingers are the only body parts that might possibly be gaining muscle strength and endurance.

The DEM System isn't an anti-exercise program nor am I proposing that you do not exercise. Exercise is great for your overall cardiovascular health but is not a major factor in weight loss. In this book, we discuss the real factors that produce rapid and sustained weight loss. I believe being physically active is important but that strenuous exercise—thirty to sixty minutes of aerobic exercise—is not a requirement for losing body fat. More physical activity throughout each day is what you need to eliminate excess body fat. So, the goal is simple: get moving and become more active, and you will enhance both your weight-loss efforts and your overall health. And getting moving does not necessarily mean going to the gym.

In this chapter, we want to discuss how you burn calories throughout the day doing everyday activities, as well as tips for achieving a higher level of fitness. You burn calories while you walk from the subway to wherever you're going, while you clean the house, while you go grocery shopping, and while you dance and have fun. What we won't focus on is going to the gym or working out as the primary method for getting physically active. If you're like me, you struggle to find time to "go somewhere to work out." Going to the gym to work out for an hour does not necessarily make us physically active. Being physically active involves the big and small movements we make throughout each day.

It's important to note that you should continue detoxifying, eating clean and balanced foods, and using the nutritional supplements discussed in Phases 1 and 2 to serve as your lifelong plan for maintaining permanent weight loss and optimal health.

Overcoming Common Excuses for Not Being Physically Active

So what's your excuse for not being physically active? First, we want to make sure that you overcome the common excuses that many people give for not being physically active. Here are the top five excuses:

I don't have enough time. Many people lead very busy and hectic lives that begin from the moment they wake up until they lie down at night to go to sleep. This causes many people to use lack of time as the reason they are not more physically active. Many men and women in the corporate world say their work schedule is too hectic. For many women, it's work, the kids, and the household that keep them too busy to get active. However, in this chapter, you'll learn easy and effective ways to get more physically active without going to the gym or finding hours of time to work out. If you have committed to getting slim and healthy, then you will need to also make the commitment to incorporate physical activity into your daily life. Just think about how much time you spend watching your favorite sitcom or reality show. If you can do that, you can find time to get active. Even if you just incorporate short bursts of activity throughout the day, it will yield you very good results. As an example, when you go to the mall or grocery store, choose the parking spot farthest away from the door to ensure that you walk a few extra steps as you go about your daily routine. Just taking a ten-minute walk will clear your head and allow you to think, refocus, and just get your mind right. So, instead of stressing about trying to find an hour to go to the gym, just try to find ten minutes here and there to move throughout each day.

I'm too tired. This one is a catch-22 situation because if you were more physically active, you'd have more energy, but until you get more physically active, you don't have the energy to get started. During this time, it is so important to gradually get physically active so that you don't push yourself too hard. The more you move, the more your metabolism and hormonal levels will improve, allowing you to get even more active. Expect your energy levels to improve first, and then over time, you'll begin to activate and strengthen your muscles with the recommendations outlined in this book. I promise you that pressing through your fatigue will help you regain the energy you need throughout each day.

I'm embarrassed. You might be embarrassed by being overweight or obese, but if you do nothing, you'll surely remain overweight and will likely gain even more weight. Use your embarrassment as motivation to do something about it. Being overweight or out of shape sends a message that you are not taking care of your body and your health. Don't hesitate to put on big baggy clothes if you feel that you want to hide your body, but by all means, get moving. You will experience so much confidence and joy when you slim down and can begin to wear more fitted clothing. You can also get moving in the comfort of your home or while at work. Getting physically active doesn't require a trip to the gym, which can be intimidating for someone really out of shape. So, if you're embarrassed, get over it! We've all been there. It's time to let your embarrassment motivate you to create a body you can be proud to show off.

I get bored exercising. I get bored doing anything I don't want to do. That's life. But I had to begin to think of getting physically active as important to my health goals. Also, I think it is imperative that your physical activity be incorporated around your hobbies or things you enjoy.

One way to eliminate the boredom of physical activity is to engage in it with a friend, an accountability buddy who can help keep you motivated and help pass the time away. Also, variety is the spice of life, so mix it up and do different activities like walking, washing the car, yoga, gardening, etc. Keep doing different activities until you find the ones that are just right for you. For additional ways to get fit and sexy at the same time, see Chapter 16.

I can't afford it. It doesn't require money to get physically active. If you look at the list of activities I recommend for getting moving, you'll notice that many of them are free, easy, and actually fun. If lack of money is an issue, then know that it is a false perception that getting fit requires a gym membership. It simply does not.

Why Physical Activity
Instead of Exercise?

There are many types of physical activity. Exercise is just one type of physical activity where you set aside a time to go work out or move your body. Exercise, which has some good health benefits, is when you set aside time for physical activity that increases your heart and lung activity while also strengthening your muscles and joints. However, physical activity is actually any kind of movement. It can be big or small movement, but it is anything that gets you on your feet and moving your body. Our goal is for you to be physically active throughout the day, even if you never go to the gym to exercise or work out. The good news is that even a minimal amount of physical activity goes a long way toward improving your health and meeting your weight-loss goals. Your goal is to move from being physically inactive to more physically active until your overall fitness level improves. You don't have to be a gym rat or bodybuilder to maintain a moderate or acceptable level of fitness.

Being physically active keeps your blood flowing and your heart pumping and keeps your mind sharp as oxygen flows to each cell in your body. Physical activity keeps your metabolism revved up throughout the day. Additionally, your muscles allow glucose (the primary source of energy from carbohydrates) to be better utilized, which will help prevent blood sugar and insulin spikes. Physical activity has also been known to improve insulin function in the body, which is especially helpful for those who have insulin resistance. A short daily walk has even been proven to reduce the risk of developing diabetes, cancer, heart disease, high blood pressure, and many other diseases.

206

Using a Step Counter

A study by Dr. James Hill found that overweight people took about 1,500 to 2,000 fewer steps a day than those who maintained a healthy weight. This means that if you can find a way to get 2,000 more steps—only about four city blocks—into your day, it could help you get to your healthy weight faster. The more steps you take, the more you speed up your metabolism and burn calories and fat. This is probably why people who live in cities maintain a healthier weight, overall, than people who live in less-dense, rural areas and drive everywhere do.

To determine how much physical activity you currently get, you may want to purchase a step counter, also called a pocket pedometer. The step counter will count how many steps you take in a given day. This will give you a picture of your current level of physical activity. A step counter is inexpensive and easy to use. You just clip it onto your skirt or pants in the morning and leave it on all day until you go to bed at night. Write down how many steps you take for about three days just following your normal daily routine.

If you are taking 5,000 steps per day or less, you are considered relatively inactive or sedentary. Your goal should be to take 7,500 steps or more per day to be considered physically active, and, of course, the more the better. One way to accomplish this is to try to add 250 steps each week until you reach a level of 7,500 or more per day. In fact, as you begin to lose weight, you'll naturally have more energy to become more physically active each week.

Of course, if your normal routine includes going to the gym, that's even better because the extra steps and movement during your workout will go toward your daily step count. The step counter keeps you motivated because it's a visual reminder to get moving throughout each day.

Tips for Getting More Physically Active

There are many great ways to get physically active without going to the gym. The goal is to make small changes in your personal and professional life that are easy to do with minimal planning and commitment. As an example, a client of mine purchased a minicycle, a set of pedals that sits on the floor or under a desk. Her goal was to use it while she sat and watched her favorite television drama. She said she kept the resistance pretty low so it wasn't too strenuous but she constantly pedaled very slowly. As a result, she lost two pounds in the first week. So she doubled the amount of time she pedaled on the minicycle while watching TV and lost three pounds the second week. It became an easy habit because she would get in a rhythm and forget she was still pedaling after a while.

Some people have gone so far as to include portable walking workstations in their office so they can either stand up or walk on a treadmill while they work or talk on the phone. You can also use the minicycle under your desk. I personally know women who have lost pounds and inches in one week just by using a minicycle while seated at their desk for an hour or two per day. If you feel uncomfortable using a portable treadmill at work, you can stand up and pace when you're on the phone and walk up and down the stairs throughout the day instead of riding the elevator.

Here are twenty-five very easy ways to simply get moving without working out or going to the gym. Please identify at least five to ten of these suggestions to incorporate into your routine, starting today. These activities can help you burn anywhere from 50 calories to 500 calories.

1. Take a brisk fifteen-minute walk at lunch. For instance, you could walk to and from a restaurant that you're visiting for lunch.

2. Work in your garden; the fresh air and natural beauty are very serene and relaxing.

3. Rake the leaves.

4. Cut your grass with a walking mower.

5. Take a yoga class, especially Bikram yoga.

6. Clean out the garage.

7. Wash the floors on your hands and knees or sweep several floors.

8. Wash your car by hand.

9. Ride your bike around the neighborhood.

10. Stroller-walk your baby.

11. Park as far as you can from the grocery store or mall and walk the remaining distance.

12. Walk more briskly in the mall while shopping.

13. While watching your favorite hour-long TV show, lift hand weights or use a minicycle to help build muscle tone and strength.

14. Pace the sidelines during your child's athletic games, which may be easy to do if you're a nervous parent!

15. Take up a new sport or hobby, like tennis, skating, bowling, bike riding, line dancing, or volleyball.

16. Get off the bus or subway one stop early and walk the remaining distance.

17. Don't email coworkers who are in your building— walk to their offices instead.

18. If you play golf, go without the golf cart.

19. Walk your dog every day.

20. Take the stairs instead of the elevator.

21. Play jump rope, double dutch, hula-hoop, or Wii with the children.

22. While on a conference call, walk around during the call.

23. Sing or play a musical instrument.

24. Turn on your favorite song and dance, dance, dance!

25. Have frequent sex, which allows you to burn about 200 calories during thirty minutes of active sex...not a bad alternative to the gym!

Moving from Physically Active to a High Level of Fitness

As you begin to get more physically active, look to advance to more cardio fitness and strength training. One way to do so is to engage in activities such as fast walking, swimming, bike riding, jogging, Zumba, or any other type of aerobic exercise. This will increase blood flow and circulation, drop blood pressure and cholesterol levels, and allow your body to better utilize blood sugar. Additionally, you want to engage the large muscle groups by incorporating more strength training. Ladies, don't get overwhelmed by the thought of lifting weights or pumping iron. You can actually build lean muscle mass without lifting weights while still achieving better balance and bone and joint strength. There are some very simple ways to activate and strengthen the muscles that can even be done in the privacy of your home. I personally like Bikram yoga because it stretches and strengthens the muscles and increases blood flow and circulation, making it a pretty complete workout routine.

After you become more physically active, you should begin to incorporate strength training into your routine, as it is key to building muscle and losing fat. Strength training uses resistance methods like free weights, weight machines, or your own body weight to build muscle and strength. Begin gradually by spending five minutes a day flexing muscles to maintain muscle mass. Since muscle mass burns more calories than fat, trying to maintain as much muscle mass as possible is very important. To actually build muscle, you can also lift weights, which is another option. However, if you don't want to lift weights and do bodybuilding, you can help keep the muscles toned and lean by using your body weight to stress your muscles a few minutes every day.

Spending just five minutes every morning flexing your muscles reminds your brain that you need your muscles and triggers the brain to burn fat instead. Short mini-muscle activities will help with muscle toning and avoid muscle atrophy.

Each day you should take five minutes to do the following mini-muscle exercises to activate and strengthen your muscles:

- Sit ups
- Pushups
- Lunges and squats
- Standing heel raises or calf raises
- Dumbbell weights to lift arms in the front and sides, as well as leg squats

Get moving and get your heart pumping by doing things that are quick, enjoyable, and easy so that "exercise" becomes a natural part of your everyday life. Exercise isn't something you have to go somewhere to do. You can and should "exercise" throughout the day to keep your metabolism supercharged.

Forget the "no pain, no gain" idea. It's not true. Easy, natural movements like walking will bring you significant gain as it relates to maintaining muscles, getting your heart rate up, and keeping your metabolism revved up throughout the day.

Why Whole-Body Vibration
Is Effective for Weight Loss

You may not have even heard of it yet, but whole-body vibration (WBV) is the exercise of the future and could likely become as common as the treadmill is today. The WBV machine uses a vibrating plate that you stand on for ten to fifteen minutes, causing rapid muscle contractions that burn calories and provide you with muscle strength that you could otherwise get by working out for an hour in the gym.

However, WBV involves no sweating or discomfort and leaves you feeling rejuvenated, calmer, and slimmer.

Many of the world's best athletes in the NFL, NHL, NBA, the Olympics, as well as Hollywood celebrities, are using WBV to lose weight, build muscle tone and bone density, relieve back pain and arthritis, improve circulation, and speed up metabolism. As a woman, I've found it to be especially beneficial for burning fat and cellulite around the thighs, hips, and buttocks.

The stimulation of whole-body vibration exercise delivers quick results that are simple yet phenomenal. WBV puts the muscles in a situation where they must expand and contract continually at a rapid rate, about twenty-five to fifty times per second, which helps to strengthen them. These contractions pump extra oxygen into the cells, which allows them to repair and regenerate quickly, resulting in amazing body transformations. Keep in mind, though, that maximum fat burning and weight loss is accomplished through WBV only when combined with proper nutrition.

The muscle contractions caused by a vibration plate will probably not build as much muscle mass as lifting weights, but unless you're a body builder, it is still very effective for maintaining muscle tone and strength.

The results of a study that took place over a few years shocked many doctors globally. Research showed that vibration exercise was four times as effective as traditional exercise for weight loss. Additionally, the group of people who used WBV kept the weight off six months after discontinuing the use of the vibration machine. Those who only dieted or either dieted with traditional exercise all gained the weight back plus some.

There are two main types of WBV machines, those that vibrate up and down using a piston-like motion (lineal) and others that vibrate from side to side like an oscillating teeter-totter (pivotal). I have personally used both, and my preference is the pivotal machines. Both machines are proven to be effective, but you should research both types if you're interested in starting a WBV routine. You can also target muscle groups by moving to different positions on the vibration machine to get even faster muscle-building results. Vibration machines are all the rage among celebrities and top athletes whose livelihood depends on their bodies being in top condition, yet they are too busy to spend hours sweating in a gym.

Summary of the Get-Moving Phase (Phase 3)

Here's a quick recap of what you need to do during this phase to get physically active and to reach a higher level of fitness.

- *Identify your top excuses for not moving.* The top five excuses as to why people don't get more physically active were discussed in this chapter. See if any of these excuses are holding you back, and if so, commit to overcoming them.

- *Measure your current level of physical activity.* To determine how much physical activity you currently get, purchase a step counter, also called a pocket pedometer, to count how many steps you take in a given day. If you don't have a step counter, just be mindful of how much you get off your feet and move around each day. Your goal should be to increase your movement each day so that you get more physically active week by week.

- *Select at least five ways to get moving.* Choose from the list of twenty-five easy ways to simply get moving without working out or going to the gym or come up with your own ideas. Incorporate your choices into your routine starting today.

- *Continue detoxifying your body, eating clean and balanced foods, and taking nutritional supplements.* All of the health-enhancing activities discussed in Phases 1 and 2 should continue to be followed during Phase 3.

In Conclusion

I want to encourage you to live life the way it was meant to be lived: active, engaged, and as a full participant. Get out of your chair, get on your feet, and go live life. Since the majority of our weight and health problems can be eliminated by following the detox guidelines, clean and balanced food recommendations, and the get-moving tips outlined in the DEM System, you can achieve optimal health. You will enjoy your new body, energy, health, and well-being. Get excited about your new life. It is not just about weight-loss—it's a journey toward optimal health and wellness. You'll love the way your body transforms, and you'll be thrilled about your results.

CHAPTER THIRTEEN

DEM System Success Stories

W e're pleased to report that so many people have experienced great success on the DEM System! Here are just a few of the many success stories we receive every week from those who are losing weight and getting healthy on the DEM System. These success stories are in their own words so you can learn what you can expect to experience while on the DEM System. It is truly a life-changing experience!

Angela's Story:

"I Lost 75 Pounds in Seven Months Without Working Out!"

The DEM System did it — saved my health, my vanity, and improved communications with my husband! After finishing the book *Lose Weight Without Dieting or Working Out*, I can honestly say I stopped ignoring my husband's attempt to talk to me about my weight. Picture someone with their hands to their ears, saying, "La La La La La La La," and you've got me.

But I digress. I started the DEM System on March 9, 2012—three days after celebrating my nineteenth wedding anniversary. At the end of the three-week Detox / Phase 1, I had lost 20.6 pounds. By October 2012, I had lost over 75 pounds! There's still more to go, but I have been celebrating what already went. I'm wearing heels again. I have a smaller stomach, an actual waistline, visible cheekbones, one chin, and a nice, long neck (now visible because of the one chin).

The weight loss is truly marvelous, but the weight loss is a boon on top of the other benefits. I have more energy, clearer skin, and a better attitude about myself. I have come a loooooooooong way in a very short period of time. They say ignorance is bliss, and it may be for some. But my ignorance was killing me, and I was living in DENIAL (Disregarding Evidence and Negating Irrefutable, Actual Logic) for years.

Regarding my size: my size 24 pants, which were supposed to be my "fat jeans," were snug, and the size 26/28 shirts weren't closing. I told a friend of mine the only time I saw a two and a zero when it came to size were together: 20. I got to see that size on my bottom half by the end of April. When I started the DEM System in March, my goal was to be in a size 18/20 pants by my fortieth birthday in August. By May, I was wearing the size 18/20 (with elastic); by June, 18s were on without any elastic. On my top, I was quickly fitting into size 24 blazers and buttoning them, not merely pulling them closed. Then I tried on a size 22 blazer in the store. I was stunned when it closed. I was so stunned, I think I cried. By mid-June, I was comfortably in a size 20 dress — from top to bottom — down from sizes 26/28. This is all WAY before my birthday. By October 2012, I was in size 14/16 tops and size 14 pants/jeans/skirts!

Also, thanks to the DEM system, I was able to fix my face. Because of the investigative aspect of monitoring my body as I reintroduced different foods, I was able to determine that my face, which was the most telling, did not react well to bread, specifically gluten and wheat. After I removed those elements from my diet on a more regular basis, my face cleared up. Woo hoo!

Reading and following the DEM System has lead to some wonderful events. During one of the most recent trips to Myrtle Beach, my husband and I actually walked on the beach. We go there often, but usually I stay in and read and look at the beach from the balcony. Now, because I have more energy, I am more willing to walk on the beach, on the boardwalk, etc. We're doing a lot more walking together. When I visited my doctor in June, she hugged me because she was proud of the improvement in my face and with the weight loss. At a recent birthday celebration for my grandmother (she turned ninety-one), I danced a good deal of the evening with my family. I wouldn't have been able to last as long as I did just four months prior. What I've learned and what I've started doing have improved the quality of life I'm living. I actually look younger, and I'm definitely healthier than I was before!

Dotta's Story:

"I Lost 20 Pounds in the Three-Week Detox Phase!"

As I sit here wondering where to start, I have tears in my eyes. No one will ever know how grateful I am to have found the DEM System. Prior to starting the DEM system, I was diagnosed with having mild osteoarthritis in both knees, with the right knee being the worst of the two. Every day and all day, I would walk around as if I were nine months pregnant. You know the wobble that pregnant women have? Well, at thirty-five years of age, I had it! Not because I was pregnant, but because my knees would hurt so badly that I would walk slowly with a limp, wobbling from side to side. The pain in my right knee would wake me up multiple times in the middle of the night. The pain was horrendous!

After being on the Detox Phase for one week, I did not feel any pain in my knees! Yes, you read that correctly! I saw a change after only one week! I could not believe how quickly I started to see results. Let me tell you, the pain never came back! Thank you, JJ!

Today, June 14, 2012, marks the twentieth day on Phase D (Detox), and so far, I have lost a whopping twenty pounds! The first week alone, I lost fourteen pounds! How can I not be excited about that? My heart is overflowing with happiness and I'm simply overjoyed. My body thanks me every day for finding this great tool! I have never lost this amount of weight in such a short time—not with any of the popular weight-loss systems or a personal trainer. I feel GREAT, too! With other weight-loss programs, I usually feel deprived, but not with the DEM system! The DEM system has taught me how to eat and what foods to choose to get my body to burn fat faster. I no longer crave sweets, including my past favorites, such as ice cream, candy bars, white carbohydrates (potato chips, rice, and macaroni and cheese), and sodas. I was addicted to sugar, but not anymore! The DEM System has changed my life, literally! I am exceptionally happy!

I have so much energy! I am no longer tired! I used to hate getting up out of a chair to do anything! Besides the pain in my knees, I used to believe I was lazy because I felt fatigued and tired all of the time. The DEM system has made me realize why I was tired. I was putting the wrong foods in my body, and because of it, my body was full of toxins. The fat that my body was trapped in felt like I had huge bricks weighing me down. I did not feel attractive, and my self-esteem certainly needed a huge boost. Because of the DEM System, I am craving fruits and vegetables and I am finding new, innovative ways to make beans! I have more self-esteem, and others have noticed it. Everyone has noticed my weight loss.

I will NEVER go back to the way I used to eat; I feel too good to go back there! I now walk with my head held high, and I walk with purpose—no wobbling included! I walk as if I AM the sexiest woman on this planet. If none of this is enough, I am receiving compliments daily. Looking at feeling healthy is what it is all about. I deserve to be healthy, and with the DEM System, I am getting closer to my goal weight each and every day!

When I started the DEM System, I wore a size 24 comfortably. NOW I am able to fit into a 20 and some 18s in my closet! I am able to wear some pants that I have not been able to wear since two summers ago! Now, THAT is PRICELESS!!! Thank you so much, JJ Smith! I thank God for you each and every day! God bless you!

Alicia's Story:

"I Lost Over 50 Pounds and My Cholesterol Dropped 50 Points!"

First, I must say thank God for JJ Smith and her new book *Lose Weight Without Dieting or Working Out*! I learned about the DEM system while listening to the radio, and immediately my friend and I decided this was something we could do. We purchased the book the same day. One of the main reasons I wanted to lose weight was that, at the time, I weighed 280 pounds and was having problems with pain and swelling in my left knee. I had just learned from my doctor that my cholesterol was too high and I would have to take medicine to lower it. I told him I didn't want to take medicine and asked if I could try diet and exercise first before being put on medicine.

Thus, my journey began (February 2012). I read your book in ONE night and began the healthy eating immediately. I must admit, I did not do the full detox program, but just began by cutting out the starch, rice, potatoes, pastas, and sugars. I immediately lost 20 pounds in the first month. In three months, my cholesterol dropped 50 points. I have lost about five inches off my waistline. By August 2012, I was at 229 pounds, down from 280 pounds. I love the way JJ explains how eating the wrong foods causes us to be overweight and how it affects our metabolism. It was also good to know that at different ages in our life, we will experience a slowdown in our metabolism, and the book explains how we can help boost our metabolism.

I thought eating healthy would be a hard challenge for me since I love fried chicken, and every Saturday morning,

I had to have fried potatoes with either bacon or sausage and three fried eggs. But I must say this has not been a challenge at all. It actually has been fun choosing exciting new healthy foods for me and my husband to eat. I cannot tell you the difference I feel now. My energy level is through the roof, and I feel great getting out of bed in the mornings. My husband and I have so much more FUN (smile) now, and I can't put into words what this has done for our relationship. I have no more knee pain or swelling at all now. I walk two miles a day with ease. JJ, all I can say is THANK YOU, THANK YOU, THANK YOU! May God continue to bless and inspire you to encourage more women. You sure have been a true encouragement to me, and I am looking forward to losing the next 29 pounds. I will be a lethal weapon then (smile). My definition of DEM — Daily Energy to Move!

Bruce's Story:

"I'm Finally Starting to See My Abs After Three Weeks!"

First, let me say THANK YOU, JJ, for writing this amazing book. It's truly a life changer and a great experience. Before the DEM system, I went to the gym three to four days a week, an hour each day, doing cardio for thirty minutes and lifting for thirty minutes, and I was weighing in at 255 pounds. I was building muscle but not losing much weight. Doing the DEM system, WITHOUT going to the gym, I am now down to 227 pounds. No matter what I did at the gym, I ended up getting big muscle mass but not losing the gut (I call it muffin top). After the three-week Detox Phase, I started seeing the abs I was looking for since high school football days.

It's working so well that I'm continuing with the Detox for five weeks. Yeah, I feel like I'm full of sludge. During the next two weeks while detoxing, I'm going to start jogging with the sauna suit and hopefully I won't pass out, but I really am ready to take it to the next level. Again, I just wanted to say thank you, JJ. I really believe in JJ and her brand and can't wait to see what's next!

Carrie's Story:

"I Lost 44 Pounds in Three Months Without Working Out!"

I am so excited, just bubbling over about the DEM system. I honestly feel like running and yelling down the street! LOL! I started the DEM System three months ago (I wanted to wait to do my review after the ninety-day mark), and right now I stand 44 pounds lighter. I cannot believe I have actually lost 44 pounds on the DEM system. My body is turning into a fat-burning machine, as I am losing three to five pounds each week on this system WITHOUT WORKING OUT! In the first two weeks, during the Detox Phase, I lost 14 pounds alone. And to be very clear, you do eat on this Detox Phase. I could never go without eating. The DEM system allows you to eat abundantly, but just different foods that help the body get healthy and burn fat!

I'm actually surprised that I have lost 44 pounds WITHOUT working out. Everyone already knows that you SHOULD work out, but sometimes you can be too heavy or too fatigued to even begin working out. It was too hard on my knees and joints, but now, starting next week, I will start walking on my treadmill that has been collecting clothes for years. LOL!

This book is simply amazing! I still think my favorite chapter is the one on ten ways to detox the body. These are some fun ways to detox that I never knew about. I learned about body brushing, which has helped smooth out that deep cellulite I had on the back of my legs. This book has so many secret tips for getting slimmer and looking and feeling better.

Here's the best part. My co-workers are stopping me, telling me how great I look, and I tell them go get this book—it is THE TRUTH! One of them is a diabetic, and I showed her the section about insulin, and she was convinced she needed this book, too. Now we have about six of us at work starting the three-week Detox Phase together. I'm gonna redo the Detox Phase with them, too, as I just love the healthy lifestyle this book promotes! I love this book... it is HIGHLY recommended to all!

Jennifer's Story:

"I Lost 16 Pounds in the Three-Week Detox Phase!"

First, let me start by saying the DEM system works and it makes sense! I had "aha" moments throughout the entire book! JJ is awesome and such an amazing mentor and motivator! I just completed my three-week Detox Phase. In the first week I lost five pounds! I remember my boyfriend telling me my face was getting skinny and there was a glow about me. I was super motivated after that!

Now let me tell you, it was tough for me that first week. Those sugar cravings were calling me! I almost gave in to those cravings, but would grab a piece of fruit instead, and the cravings would fade. By week two, I had lost another six pounds and was feeling pretty amazing, my cravings were gone, and I honestly began to crave fruit and salads. I remember having lunch with a friend who had a greasy burger, fries, and soda. It didn't bother me at all. I had my lavish salad and I was fine. I couldn't believe it!! By week three, I had lost another five pounds! So my total weight lost for the three-week Detox has been 16 pounds!

Let me tell you, I got my confidence back, and it's soaring! I celebrate non-scale victories like my favorite jeans now fitting looser and being able to comfortably cross my legs. I can now button up one of my favorite coats. I can wrap the bath towel around my body. Most importantly, I have asthma, and sometimes I have to remind myself to take my medication because I'm breathing so much better! My sleep is even better and more restful! All the benefits that come along with being on the system are incredible! These are my immediate victories after completing the three-week Detox. I'm not going to say it was easy. It was NOT for the first week or so; actually, it was one of the hardest things I've done in my life, trying to break the addictions, but it works if you stay committed, and it gets better. You soon begin to realize you can do this and win. You begin to realize you have the power to get yourself back!

The DEM system has been life changing. Although I want to be rid of this unwanted weight (and I will), it's not about fast weight loss. For me, it's no longer about a quick fix, it's about me evolving, changing from the inside out—and changing my relationship with food! I had no clue as to what healthy eating truly meant until this book, even with me being a healthcare professional! This book teaches you how to be aware and make the right choices. I'm a label reader now! I'm conscious about every single thing I put in my body, and what I love is it's not a diet. DEM is a life change. This is the only thing I have found that I can honestly do for a lifetime. In fact, I'm back on the DEM three-week phase because I loved the results and how I felt, so why not stay here for a while? It works. I'm a testament to that. It works if you stay committed. Stick to it—you've got everything to lose! I'm getting my sexy back.

Todd's Story:

"The DEM System Gave Me the Six-Pack Abs I've Always Wanted!"

This book helped me experience how good I could feel by eliminating bad foods from my diet during the Detox Phase. I now feel more alert, mentally sharp, and I don't have the highs and lows that I used to experience each day. I've never considered myself "really" overweight, but I'm 44 years old and, like most men, I have always dreamed of having a six-pack. I have worked out off and on my entire life, but I could never achieve that elusive six-pack until I discovered the DEM system. I lost 14 pounds in three weeks and am constantly looking at or taking pics of my abs. My abs look better now than they did when I was 21 years old!

Whitley's Story:

"I Lost 17 Pounds in Three Weeks and Still Got to Eat!"

I bought this book and read it in one day. Let me first start off by saying I have read every popular diet book in the world, but I must say I have NEVER learned so much about why I have been fat my entire life until I read this book. The book is truly AMAZING. I'm not even gonna start by telling you how much weight I lost, although that has me jumping for joy. I want people to understand something that's changed for the very first time, something NO other diet book did for me. I've changed my lifestyle. I don't crave unhealthy foods; I don't want them. I'm not trying to avoid them like when you're "on a diet." I truly desire salads and fresh fruits, nuts, and seeds. My mind has changed, my cravings have changed, and my body is thanking me for it.

The book starts with a Detox Phase and has you avoid unhealthy foods, do supplements, and take colon cleansers for twenty-one days. This was the part that changed my cravings and eating habits. The Detox Phase was easy for me because I got to eat...and eat abundantly. But it was just different stuff than I was used to eating. The book helped me to understand I was a sugar addict. I was addicted to pop, candy, cakes, and energy drinks, and I hardly ever ate anything healthy. This is why I always gained the weight back after my diets; I never really broke the addictions and always went back to unhealthy eating. After the three weeks on the Detox Phase, I was delighted to be down 17 pounds.

I just didn't lose 17 pounds in the first three weeks. In fact, there are many diets where you can lose weight, but the trick is how to keep the weight off. Unlike any other diet I've tried (and geeesh, I've tried them all), I am feeling better than I have in about twenty years. I am 49 years old, was tired, fatigued, unhappy, and had dull skin and hair. I thought this is just what happens as you get older. But my co-workers are telling me I look good. They say I look slimmer, younger. People are noticing, which is great, but I tell you the information in this book has literally made me feel twenty years younger. I'm sleeping better, I feel more solid, happier. I just LOVE the way I'm feeling and, for the first time in a long time, I CANNOT wait for summer to get here! Bring it on!

Carolyn's Story:

"The DEM System is Clear, Concise, and Makes Perfect Sense!"

JJ's system of Detox, Eat, and Move (DEM) is easy to follow with clear instructions. She admits the first three-week Detox Phase is the hardest, as you work to detoxify and cleanse the body through avoiding certain foods and doing other detox methods, such as digestive cleansers and green drinks. In this phase, you flush out toxins that cause weight gain and re-train your taste buds so you can establish healthier eating habits.

As a woman, my favorite section was all the information geared just for the ladies on how to avoid menopausal weight gain, as well as tips to get rid of cellulite and belly fat and other issues that women struggle with.

229

What I loved most about this book is that I've read bits and pieces about eating healthy, detoxifying, and weight loss, in general, but never have I read it ALL consolidated in one place. JJ lays it all out for you in the easy-to-follow DEM System. I wish I had a binder or notebook so I could take all the shopping lists to the grocery store. There are so many foods and supplements that she recommends, and I need to carry this book with me as I go shopping. The book is jam-packed with great suggestions WITHOUT crazy fad diets, calorie counting (which JJ says is useless), boxed foods, or extreme workouts... it's just great, solid info!

Megan's Story:

"This Book Is the Bible for Healthy Living!"

I must admit that this book has changed my life! OH MY GAWD! I wanted to lose weight when I bought this book, and I did, but WOW, this book has become my bible for healthy living. I never learned so much about my body and health EVER! The book has changed my whole way of eating, and detoxing has really cleared up my adult acne, indigestion, and bloating. I really struggled with those things, but today I feel great!

I have been on the DEM system for two months and I have lost about 21 pounds and I don't know how many inches. My birthday is coming up soon, and I will be fine at 40! It feels so good TO LOOK SO GOOD! YAY ME! It's so amazing how much weight I lost without having to work out, and I lost so much belly fat. I'm quite happy about that.

One last thing is there is a really powerful chapter called Motivation for a New Body and a New You. It was so moving, as it talked about self-love being key to maintaining your healthy, ideal weight. Powerful, powerful chapter...worth the price of the book alone!

I SO HIGHLY RECOMMEND this book. I even bought five copies for my momma and girlfriends and wrapped them as gifts! Everyone I know and love MUST have this book!

Laura's Story:

"As a Personal Trainer, I Recommend This Book to All My Clients!"

As a personal fitness trainer, I wanted to not like this book because of the title. But the truth is, the book is the real deal. The book discourages "diets" and instead offers some great tips for simply eating healthy and smart. I ABSOLUTELY love that!

The book teaches a DEM System (Detox, Eat, Move), and it is right on point, especially since the "move" part includes ways to get physically active, which includes exercise. It's just that the book says you don't have to maintain an exercise regimen to get results, but it still encourages everyone to get more physically active. If the book had discouraged exercising, I would have strongly disliked it. It's actually the most comprehensive book on weight loss I have ever read. There is not a single question that you might have about weight loss that she does not answer. I've begun using the DEM System with my clients, also. The tips throughout the book will DEFINITELY help you get slimmer AND healthier at the same time. I am a HUGE fan of JJ Smith and this book!

Marcia's Story:

"I Lost 17 Pounds in Less Than Five Weeks and Have Not Worked Out at All!"

The DEM System is AMAZING!! I started the DEM system on April 30th and was very skeptical because I've tried so many things to lose weight and can't seem to get where I want to be. I would love to meet JJ in person and thank her and give her a huge hug. She introduced me to a new way of life. This is not a DIET, it's a new way of living and taking care of yourself and your body.

I lost 17 pounds in less than five weeks on the DEM system and have not worked out at all. I usually use my stationery bike and other equipment, but have not at all these past five weeks. I know I lost a few inches because all my clothing fits differently. I'm going to start using my stationery bike and doing crunches to see if I can escalate my weight loss.

I'm getting married in September and want to look amazing for my fiancé. I initially started this for my wedding, but I don't think I will ever go back to eating the way I used to. If I can announce it to the world, I would: JJ Smith's DEM system is the only way to live your life healthy and naturally! Thank you from the bottom of my heart, JJ!

Tennille's Story:

"I Lost Six Pounds in Six Days and Noticed a Smaller Midrift!"

Thank you so much for sharing with the rest of us! I

just finished reading your wonderful book (and sent copies to my mother and two friends) and am on day eight of the Detox Phase. I can't believe I have gone without sugar for eight days and I feel just great! Ecstatic! I definitely had toxic overload when starting this program and have been incorporating liver-friendly foods that you mentioned in your book. I have already noticed a smaller midsection. In the first six days, I had already lost six pounds!

Your wealth of knowledge is so on point and true and makes complete sense. I am in the healthcare field and you are so right how so many ailments caused by poor eating habits are "treated" with prescription meds instead of detoxifying the body and then giving it the healthy, natural nutrition it craves. Your book is clearly life changing, and I am so excited to continue to see how my body positively responds. As one example, I used to have true caffeine addiction for years. I now notice how every morning after having my "green drink," I feel a real burst of energy and mental clarity that lasts for hours! I could go on and on but just wanted to chime in and say thank you so much for sharing. You could have kept this all to yourself, but you didn't! Thank you for being a blessing to so many!"

Cheri's Story:

"My Acne is Clearing and My Skin is Soft and Radiant!"

Let me begin by expressing my gratitude to you for your book. I absolutely love it! Being an avid reader, I come across many books that I love and recommend to others because I find the information within to be somewhat informational or delightful. It is very rare that I find a book that actually produces results.

I am sharing my gratitude to you because the insight and knowledge that you have shared through your books have accomplished results that the doctors and dermatologist couldn't do! Not only am I more attentive and aware of my health, for the first time I am gaining confidence and a newfound appreciation for my life, my body, and my face—and no amount of money can replace what I am experiencing now.

I have battled with acne for more than twenty years and have tried numerous products, and all brought forth disappointment. My acne is clearing, my skin is more soft and radiant, and others are also commenting instead of looking away awkwardly.

PART 4

Issues for Women Only

Issues for Women Only

Research has confirmed that it is more difficult for women to lose weight than men because women's bodies are simply more efficient at storing fat. Therefore, women have to be much more deliberate about losing body fat and managing their weight. The DEM System allows you to make some key changes to your diet and lifestyle that help you discover a slimmer, sexier, healthier you!

In this section, we'll explore some natural ways to help you achieve your most beautiful, youthful, and energetic self. We'll discuss unique issues affecting women, such as dealing with menopausal weight gain and aging skin, and provide some fun ways to get fit and sexy!

CHAPTER FOURTEEN

Health, Beauty, and Vibrance for Women Over Forty

I believe that natural, healthy eating is the secret to inner and outer beauty. When you eat natural, organic foods, you simply look and feel better and younger. Once you eat in a manner that keeps your cells clean and healthy, you will begin to look radiant, despite your age. Human beings are designed to eat a diet primarily made up of fruits, vegetables, seeds, and nuts. With these types of natural, healthy foods, our bodies flourish and receive all of the necessary nutrients to keep our bodies toxin-free and looking our most beautiful. Many begin the DEM System to simply lose weight but they end up noticing a dramatic improvement in their health, with renewed energy and a decrease in their ailments and illnesses.

When you begin the DEM System, one of the first places you'll see changes is in the quality of your skin. Healthy eating and living will remove years from your face, eliminate wrinkles, fade age spots, and give you a "second youth." Your skin will become supple, and acne will clear up. Your eyes will become brighter and begin to sparkle. The dark circles and puffiness will diminish as well as the yellowness in the whites of your eyes. On the inside of your body, your cells will become rejuvenated as well, causing your organs to function more efficiently. The journey through detox fasting and cleansing is not only good for weight loss, but it is also a pathway to a second youth, greater mental clarity, and balanced moods.

Top Five Foods to Slow Aging, Fight Wrinkles, and Keep Skin Youthful

Have you noticed that your skin has begun to look dull and tired? Have you noticed a few fine lines and wrinkles? Has your youthful glow begun to fade? There are natural ways to provide your skin with the nutrients it needs to help you have healthier, brighter, and younger-looking skin! The following five foods will slow the aging of your skin and diminish the wrinkles and fine lines.

- *Green leafy veggies.* These foods contain vitamin A and beta-carotene and help you have bright and smooth skin. As far as food goes, it doesn't get much better than green leafy vegetables, such as kale, spinach, collards, etc. Vitamin A helps your skin produce more fresh, new cells and get rid of the old ones, reducing dryness and keeping your face looking bright and young.

- *Citrus fruits.* Vitamin C, a prime ingredient in tons of beauty creams, aids in the production of collagen. Once you turn thirty-five, collagen starts to break down, leaving your skin saggy. Citrus fruits, like oranges, lemons, grapefruits, and even tomatoes, contain vitamin C, and eating them helps you have smooth and tight/taut skin.

- *Berries (especially blueberries and blackberries).* These delicious berries keep skin looking younger longer and help fight wrinkles. Berries are considered by many experts to be one of the highest food sources of antioxidants, which target free radicals that can wreak havoc on skin cells. Blueberries, in particular, are good for fighting aging, and the best are organic wild blueberries. Fresh or frozen blueberries are very good options also.

- *Nuts and seeds.* These foods contain vitamin E, which helps you have soft, youthful-looking skin. Incorporate more of the easily digestible seeds and nuts, like almonds, pistachios, walnuts, flaxseed, pumpkin seeds, sesame seeds, and sunflower seeds, into your diet to help provide that youthful, soft skin.

- *Seafood.* The omega-3 fatty acids and zinc in seafood reduce dryness and inflammation of the skin. Most of us have heard that fish can be really good for overall health—it's a primary component in what's known as the "Mediterranean diet." Many types of fish and shellfish can also work wonders for the skin, especially oysters, salmon, and tuna.

Supplements for Youthful, Glowing Skin

You can supplement your diet with certain vitamins and other ingredients that specifically support healthy, radiant hair, skin, and nails.

- *Vitamin C* is a natural Botox. Women with higher dosages of vitamin C in their diet were 11 percent less likely to develop wrinkles.

- *Vitamin E* restores moisture to the skin and slows the aging of skin cells. Green leafy vegetables and nuts are good sources of vitamin E.

- *Vitamin A* also helps to keep wrinkles away. The best forms of vitamin A are its derivatives, such as retinoids like Retin-A and the more moisturizing Renova. They work by removing the top layer of dead skin cells while generating collagen in the skin. Collagen is the skin's structural fiber, and as we get older, it breaks down, creating fine lines and larger pores. Skincare experts disagree on all sorts of things, but most of them consider retinoids to be a miracle skin saver. Retinoid treatments can also help with acne, age spots, sun damage, and freckles.

- *Niacin* (vitamin B3) is used for a variety of skin problems, including acne, inflammation, sagging skin, and dull skin tone. Regular use of niacin will help to reduce these ailments.

- *Omega-3 fatty acids* are "healthy fats" that help maintain cell membranes so that they efficiently allow water and nutrients in and keep toxins out. They also help to protect skin against sun damage.

You don't necessarily have to take each of these as individual supplements. There are multivitamins targeted for healthy hair, skin, and nails that contain many of these ingredients.

Reduce Cellulite and Sagging Skin

Cellulite is the dimpled accumulation of stored fat on our thighs and buttocks caused by a sluggish lymphatic system. The lymphatic system is a secondary circulatory system underneath the skin that rids the body of toxic wastes, bacteria, and dead cells. By cleansing the liver and lymphatic system, you help rid the body of fatty deposits—the key to diminishing cellulite.

Another cause of cellulite is loose or weakening skin and connective tissues that are unable to keep the fat tissues contained within their compartments. As the fat tissues or deposits escape through weakened connective strands, they create the dimply, pebbly effect known as cellulite. So strengthening the skin and muscles is a great preventive measure for cellulite. Foods containing protein help to firm up muscles that can keep fat stores in place and reduce the dimpled effect of cellulite.

Here are some specific tips for reducing cellulite:

- *Body brushing.* Body-brushing improves circulation, removes dead skin layers, and encourages cell renewal for a much smoother-textured skin. This process also eliminates toxins by stimulating the lymphatic system. (See Chapter 5 for details on how and when to do your body brushing.)

- *Drink green tea.* Green tea burns fat really well, especially stubborn fat areas like cellulite. I try to drink two cups per day.

- *Eating lean proteins.* When your body lacks protein, your facial skin, and the skin on your arms and legs, begins to sag due to lost collagen. Those with thinning hair and too many wrinkles for their age, or puffy eyes, may lack protein. Your muscles, hair, nails, skin, and eyes are made of protein. It is necessary for tissue repair, and every cell in our body needs protein to maintain its life and replace dead cells. If you follow the guidelines in this book (i.e., the amount of protein to eat) daily, you will get the sufficient amount that your body needs every day. However, if you are very active or weightlifting, then you should increase your protein intake, typically done by drinking protein powder shakes to repair and rebuild muscle.

Reduce Belly Fat for a Sexy Waistline

There are some unique challenges we women face when it comes to losing weight. One of the questions most commonly asked of me is, "How do I get rid of belly fat?" Let's discuss belly fat in general and then discuss the following strategies for achieving a slimmer waistline:

- Get rid of toxins

- Eliminate stress

- Treat estrogen dominance

If we look at people with flat stomachs and six-packs, they look like a picture of good health, fitness, and strength. A flat, tight stomach is a sign that someone is in control of her body and in control of her health. Most people will admit to wanting a thinner waistline, and this is not shallow at all. Tight, sexy abs are rated the sexiest body part by many men and women. When you appear in control of your health, it's a sign to the world that you are not only a highly motivated, disciplined, and healthy person, but that you are an attractive and desirable mate as well.

We all know what belly fat is; we see it every day when we walk out of the house. Belly fat, known as visceral fat, is located behind your abdominal wall and surrounds your internal organs. Visceral fat typically shows as the belly fat/spare tire around the waist and mid-section. Even thin people can begin to store excess weight around the stomach and midsection. Visceral fat contains toxins and substances that are harmful to our health and can affect the nervous system and the endocrine (hormonal) system, which ends up affecting metabolism and appetite.

Most people do not know that belly fat is the most dangerous fat on the body. Because of where it's located around the delicate organs, it has the potential to destroy good health, or worse yet, kill you. Because belly fat resides within striking distance of your heart, liver, and other organs, it is to blame for many health conditions. According to a 2006 study published in the journal *Obesity*, visceral fat is a significant predictor of early death. In other words, visceral fat means you have an increased risk for a shortened life. Even if you removed visceral fat via liposuction, it may cause you to look physically better, but it does little for improving your health because the dangers of visceral fat would still exist for you. The good news is that even a minimal amount of physical activity and dietary changes will go a long way in shrinking visceral fat.

Get Rid of Toxins to Decrease Belly Fat

Studies have shown that exposing yourself to an excessive amount of environmental toxins increases belly fat. Thus, a very effective way to address this visceral fat/belly fat is to eliminate toxins from the body. Follow the detoxification methods provided in Chapter 5 to eliminate toxins, thereby reducing belly fat.

Eliminate Stress to Reduce Belly Fat

Stress may be another factor that affects belly fat.

When you are stressed, your body releases a hormone called cortisol (also known as stress hormone). Studies have shown that when cortisol is released into the bloodstream, you become less sensitive to leptin, the hormone that tells your brain you are full. When this happens, you tend to eat more and more and begin to crave sugar. And fat caused by stress tends to get stored in the belly.

To reduce the stress in your life, follow these tips:

- *Place "happy photos" at work and in your car (like on the visor)*. When you look at them, they will immediately take you to a happy place, causing stress levels to decrease.

- *Make love*. The more we make love, the more endorphins our brains release. These "neuro-hormones" that are released in the brain act as natural painkillers and help to alleviate anxiety.

- *Schedule "playtime" with your significant other or children*. Doing fun things like miniature golf, bowling, and seeing a movie can take your mind off your stress.

- *Smile often and laugh a lot*. If you have a favorite comedian, include a CD in your car to listen to as you drive to and from work. Or watch movies that make you laugh out loud. Or listen to music that calms you down or makes you sing along.

- *Get a massage*. Deep-pressure massage stimulates the nerves that cause levels of the stress hormone cortisol to diminish. Research has also shown that those who *give* massages reduce their own levels of stress hormones.

- *Get moving.* It is well documented that regular physical activity or exercise helps to alleviate stress and raise body temperature, which helps the body prepare for sleep. There's strong evidence that moderate exercise like brisk walking activates the "feel good" neurotransmitters dopamine and serotonin, which reduce the symptoms of depression.

- *Build better relationships.* The biggest enemy of good health is stress. The biggest enemy of stress is solid relationships with other people. So show more respect and compassion to other people, even more than you feel they deserve. This might seem to hurt you in the short term, but it is a sure investment in the long term.

- *Sleep more.* Too many Americans are sleep-deprived. However, I can honestly say I am not one of them. I am a huge fan of sleep. I get my eight hours of sleep every night, and if I fall short one night, I make up for it over the weekend. Sleep is the body's way of recharging the system and is the easiest yet most underrated activity to heal the body. Sleep also helps to eliminate puffy red eyes and dark circles. There isn't anything that can compensate for lack of sleep. Lack of sleep accelerates wear and tear, accelerating aging, and pushes the body out of its natural balance and rhythm. Short-changing sleep time or going to bed stressed interferes with the best time for losing those extra pounds. So be sure to relax or meditate before going to sleep. Relaxing causes cortisol levels to drop, which will in turn help your body burn more calories. In short, getting enough sleep helps you burn more calories at night and during the day.

Treat Estrogen Dominance to Reduce Belly Fat and Bloating

If you are like me and have been frustrated with extra fat and bloating around your waist and abdomen, you will also be pleased to know that sometimes those extra pounds have little to do with how many crunches you're doing or how much less food you're eating and everything to do with a shift in hormones that happens with almost everyone over the age of thirty-five. Excess belly fat is often due to a hormonal imbalance called estrogen dominance, which can occur primarily in women but sometimes in men, also. If you don't address estrogen dominance, your stubborn belly fat will likely remain and be impossible to lose no matter how much you cut down on calories or work out.

The good news is that estrogen dominance can be treated, and once your hormones have been properly balanced, the extra fat around your waist will begin to melt away. For a more detailed explanation of estrogen dominance, see Chapter 15.

In women, and oftentimes men, higher estrogen levels cause the body to store fat around the waist and abdomen area. More specifically, in women, estrogen dominance causes fat to be stored around the stomach, waist, hips, and thighs, causing us to look round or pear-shaped once we get in our forties. For men, it causes them to have the fat belly that looks like a spare tire around their waist.

The three best ways to address belly fat caused by estrogen dominance are:

- Eating a clean and balanced diet, as discussed in Chapter 11. This will ensure that you avoid foods that cause estrogen-mimicking toxins to circulate in the body.

- Using natural hormone replacement therapy, also called bio-identical hormone replacement therapy (BHRT), to restore hormonal balance (see Chapter 14 for more details).

- Taking nutritional supplements that eliminate excess estrogen circulating in the body, thereby providing the hormonal balance required to lose unwanted fat, namely belly fat (see Chapter 14 for more details).

Women who address these three factors successfully relieve their symptoms of estrogen dominance, namely that bloated belly, within one to two months. For me personally, to have my stomach literally deflate from bloated to flat happened within a few short weeks.

Most women over forty begin to experience some of the trouble areas we've discussed in this chapter: belly fat, cellulite, and fine lines and wrinkles. Now you have some real strategies to deal with the trouble spots and reverse the aging process so that you will look and feel more youthful.

CHAPTER FIFTEEN

Stop Weight Gain During Perimenopause and Menopause

I f you're over thirty-five, you may have begun to notice a few extra pounds around your waist, hips, thighs, and butt. You may not have changed your eating habits or exercise routine but may still be unable to maintain your weight. You should be happy to know that you are definitely not alone.

Weight gain, along with overall change in body shape, is normal and should be expected. Over 90 percent of women gain weight between the ages of thirty-five and fifty-five. The average weight gain during this period of perimenopause and menopause is fifteen to twenty pounds, around one to two pounds per year, and the earlier you move into perimenopause the more extreme and rapid the weight gain will be. It's not just that you gain weight, it's also how the weight tends to be distributed around your waistline, belly, thighs, hips, and butt area that makes your body appear to be more round and less curvy. As your estrogen levels decline, they also affect the production of collagen, which results in drier, thinner skin, saggy tissue, and lack of muscle tone—all factors that contribute to a change in your body shape.

Even if you eat in the same manner as you did for years, you can expect weight gain as you get closer to the perimenopause/menopause years. Weight gain, especially around the mid-section, as well as soft, jiggly arms, hips, and thighs, are all unfortunate realities of getting older. I have personally experienced this frustration and know many other women who have experienced this undesirable weight gain. Unfortunately, our bodies become naturally insulin-resistant as we age, which makes us more inclined to store fat, especially around the waist. Additionally, our ovaries are beginning to produce less estrogen during perimenopause, which causes the body's fat cells to try to produce more estrogen. While fat cells are not the primary source of estrogen production in the body, they do produce estrogen. However, once you achieve hormonal balance, you can get back to a body that burns fat instead of storing it.

Weight gain in this stage of life is due to fluctuating hormones, but the good news is that you can achieve a better hormone balance. You do not have to accept getting heavier and heavier as you age, and yes, you can lose those extra pounds.

Understanding Perimenopause and Menopause

Menopause is the time in a woman's life when her menstruation stops and she is no longer fertile (i.e., no longer able to become pregnant). Perimenopause is the stage that precedes menopause, and it may last for many years. It's the transition from normal menstrual periods to no periods at all.

Perimenopausal women can be emotional, moody, and irritable because they are still getting a period, albeit it is very irregular—sometimes heavy and sometimes very light. This rather severe state of hormonal imbalance causes hormonal surges and symptoms. This stage officially marks the beginning of hormonal decline, resulting in symptoms such as weight gain, mood swings, hot flashes, sleeplessness, lack of sex drive, fatigue, and irritability. Women in their late thirties and early forties may already be beginning this transition, and as their bodies experience hormonal confusion, unexplained symptoms begin to pop up. (When I went through it, I got seasonal allergies for the first time in my life.)

Even though perimenopause and menopause are normal processes that all women will go through, experiencing the symptoms associated with them can be minimized or avoided altogether. If you are in this stage of life, you have to be diligent about finding the right doctor who will understand what is really going on in your body. Most doctors will simply treat the symptoms; very few tie all of them together and address the root cause of the problem. The underlying problem is hormone loss, and the sooner you replace these hormones, the better you will look and feel. No one is going to be as committed to doing this as you. Know that perimenopause is your wake-up call to take action to restore your health back to a state where you felt balanced, youthful, and energetic.

By the time you get to menopause, you should already be so actively balancing your hormones that this next transition in life should not have to feel painful and depressing, and you should experience fewer symptoms of hot flashes, night sweats, mood swings, and other menopausal symptoms. You will begin even more hormonal decline, but you'll also be able to continue tweaking your hormones so you feel balanced and healthy.

It's important to research and understand what happens with hormonal decline in each transition phase of your life, from perimenopause to menopause and beyond.

Three Key Sex Hormones That Affect Weight Gain

There are three key sex hormones that can become imbalanced as you age. Fluctuating hormonal levels of estrogen, progesterone, and testosterone cause weight gain, mood swings, irregular menstrual cycles, and many other symptoms that we'll discuss in this chapter.

Estrogen

Estrogen, produced by the ovaries, is what transforms us from girls into women. It gives us our curves and helps regulate our passage through fertility and menstruation. Estrogen occurs in the body in three compounds: estradiol (most potent estrogen), estrone (dominant estrogen after menopause), and estriol (weakest form of estrogen, at its highest levels during pregnancy). Estrogen stimulates growth in breasts, ovaries, and the uterus. Both men and women have estrogen, but women have much higher levels of it.

Estrogen is one of the two main hormones produced in the ovaries. The other, progesterone, is produced primarily in the second half of a woman's menstrual cycle. When women reach their thirties and forties, it is very common for the balance between the two hormones to shift heavily toward estrogen, causing a condition known as estrogen dominance, resulting in night sweats, depression, fatigue, weight gain, anxiety, blood sugar imbalance, low sex drive, dry skin and hair, cellulite, and brain fog. Too much estrogen in the body also causes salt and water retention, making us look bloated, flabby, and soft. However, the estrogen and progesterone levels can be balanced to relieve these symptoms.

Progesterone

Your body secretes progesterone every month after an egg is released. During times of high levels of progesterone, the body burns 100 to 300 more calories per day than it does during times of high levels of estrogen. Progesterone also helps to reduce bloating and uterine fibroids, improves libido, and boosts mental clarity.

As I stated earlier, when your progesterone levels overall start to drop, estrogen dominance sets in, and you may experience early symptoms of menopause, known as perimenopause. When you have low levels of progesterone, you may also experience premenstrual syndrome and possibly depression. The sudden appearance of abdominal fat, in particular, is a sign that the body's internal hormonal ratio of progesterone to estrogen is unbalanced.

A primary goal of hormone balancing is to restore the balance between estrogen and progesterone to create harmony and balance in our body. When estrogen and progesterone are properly balanced, these two hormones help the body burn fat, boost metabolism, and relieve the symptoms of estrogen dominance.

Luckily, there are foods that enhance your progesterone levels, allowing you to better metabolize fat and sleep better. The B vitamin family, in particular B6, is key to enhancing progesterone levels. You can get B vitamins in meat, poultry, fish, beans, and some fruits and vegetables, like bananas, avocados, spinach, and tomatoes. Another key nutrient that will help progesterone production is magnesium, found in dark green leafy vegetables, eggs, meat, seeds, nuts, and beans. Fortunately, these foods high in magnesium will also keep your liver healthy. Poor liver function causes hormonal imbalances, and in particular, suppresses progesterone.

Testosterone

Testosterone often is overlooked when women are dealing with perimenopause and menopausal symptoms. However, women with low testosterone levels experience fatigue, weakness, low energy, low motivation, muscle atrophy, and a lowered sex drive.

Men naturally make 50 percent more testosterone than women; however, it is a vital hormone in women also. Many women are surprised to hear that testosterone is actually produced in small amounts by the ovaries and the adrenal glands. This hormone supports a woman's body by helping it to maintain its energy levels, muscle tone, vaginal elasticity, sex drive, and overall vitality.

Between the ages of thirty-five and fifty-five, women typically lose about 50 percent of their testosterone, and this too contributes to unpleasant symptoms. During perimenopause, which can begin as early as thirty-five, ovulation becomes irregular, and both progesterone and testosterone levels begin to decline. In some situations, a woman may have high levels of testosterone; when this occurs, she can experience acne or other skin breakouts, the growth of facial hair, and weight gain.

As we age, we all experience a decline in hormone levels. Women lose 30 percent of their estrogen by age fifty, 75 percent of their progesterone, and 50 percent of their testosterone between ages thirty-five and fifty. Both progesterone and estrogen then continue to decline sharply after menopause. The reality is that we all experience the symptoms of hormonal decline. However, there are some ways that we can maintain a better hormonal balance and minimize these unpleasant symptoms.

Estrogen Dominance Is the Primary Hormonal Imbalance Causing Weight Gain

When estrogen levels remain high in the body relative to progesterone, the result is a condition known as estrogen dominance. The primary symptoms of estrogen dominance are weight gain (especially around the abdomen, hips, and thighs), sluggish metabolism, mood swings, irregular periods, and bloating. I know of estrogen dominance all too well, and every one of these symptoms was very real and very frustrating to me.

Estrogen dominance also causes increased bloating and water retention—which may not be the result of more fat but still makes you look heavier and causes your blood sugar to fluctuate, which increases your appetite and slows your metabolism. When women are menstruating, this bloating occurs right around the menstrual cycle. When women no longer have periods and are not producing progesterone, the bloating will be a constant problem. Progesterone acts as a natural diuretic. Progesterone also encourages the body to use calories from food for energy; without enough progesterone, the body is compromised in its ability to metabolize calories, and the calories get stored as fat in the body.

Estrogen dominance can cause insulin resistance (see Chapter 6 for more information), which causes insulin to be released more often than it is needed. This extra release of insulin causes the body to crave sugar and to store fat. However, balancing estrogen and progesterone levels helps to regulate the release of insulin. In both sexes, estrogen dominance is thought to be one of the leading causes of breast, uterine, and prostate cancer.

Contrary to the popular belief that estrogen is a "female" hormone, men can also be estrogen dominant. One possible cause of estrogen dominance is exposure to environmental estrogens, and men are exposed to the same ones as women. Men who show signs of estrogen dominance are typically over the age of forty and experience weight gain around the middle, hair loss, development of breasts, and fatigue.

The "thickening" of women's bodies and the "softening" of men's bodies are often related to excess estrogen. When in excess, estrogen promotes the growth of estrogen-sensitive tissues, known as "stubborn fat" because they are highly resistant to fat burning. Even if you eat less and exercise, this doesn't help remove the estrogen-sensitive fat. You get caught in a vicious cycle as excess estrogen promotes fat gain; the enlarged estrogen-sensitive fat tissue produces more estrogen within its cells, which then promotes more fat gain, and so on.

Common symptoms of estrogen dominance include:

- Stubborn fat/weight gain around stomach area, hips, thighs, and butt
- Water retention/bloating
- Tender breasts
- Low libido
- Problematic PMS/menstrual cramps
- Dry skin/vaginal dryness
- Mood swings or irritability
- Hot flashes/night sweats
- Insomnia
- Brain fog or "fuzzy thinking"
- Irregular periods or heavy or long-lasting periods
- Fatigue
- Depression or low motivation
- Cyclical migraine headaches
- Infertility or frequent miscarriage
- Fibrocystic breasts
- Uterine fibroids
- Endometriosis
- Low-thyroid symptoms
- Polycystic ovary syndrome (PCOS)
- Breast cancer

What Causes Estrogen Dominance?

There are three likely causes of estrogen dominance. Let's take a look at each one.

- As you age, your hormonal levels begin to fluctuate, and your body can produce too much estrogen relative to the progesterone levels in your body.

- Taking hormone replacement therapy (HRT) or birth control pills for many years.

- Regular exposure to xenoestrogens, manmade compounds that mimic the effects of natural estrogens in the body. Xenoestrogens are chemicals in pesticides, plastics, soaps, household cleaning products, and even car exhausts that look and act enough like natural estrogens that the body mistakenly accepts them as estrogen. Many xenoestrogens are fat soluble and pass through the skin easily. They accumulate over time, resulting in excessive amounts of estrogen circulating in the bloodstream.

Bio-identical Hormone Replacement Therapy (BHRT) to Naturally Balance Hormones

The good news is that bio-identical hormone replacement therapy (BHRT) can solve the problem of estrogen dominance by allowing you to increase the amount of progesterone in your body. The result will be a reduction in or the elimination of many of the symptoms of perimenopause/menopause. But since BHRT is not very widely accepted by the medical establishment and is considered "alternative medicine," you will have to do some research to find a good doctor qualified to prescribe it. Believe me, it is well worth the search.

Bio-identical hormones are hormones derived from plants, usually soybeans or wild yams, through a biochemical process that ensures that the molecular structure is identical to the hormones women make in their bodies. Synthetic hormones are not identical in either structure or activity to the natural hormones they emulate. The body can't distinguish bio-identical hormones from the ones your ovaries produce, so they fit perfectly into the hormone receptors like a lock and key. Hormones work like a key in a lock. Bio-identical hormones fit that lock perfectly. Synthetic hormones fit some, but not all, of the hormone receptor (lock) sites. This causes synthetic hormones to have more side effects than bio-identical hormones because of a poor lock and key fit. Bio-identical hormones (key) fit perfectly into the hormone receptors (lock), causing the body to recognize and accept bio-identical hormones just as it would recognize and accept naturally occurring human hormones, making it both effective and safe.

The great appeal of bio-identical hormones is that they are natural, and our bodies can metabolize them as they were designed to do, minimizing side effects. Synthetic hormones are quite strong and often produce intolerable side effects. The other important factor is that bio-identical hormones can be matched individually to each woman's hormonal needs, something that's close to impossible to do with mass-produced synthetic products. According to a study published in *The Journal of the American Medical Association*, synthetic hormones were found to increase a woman's risk of breast cancer, heart disease, blood clots, and stroke. Studies show that bio-identical hormones are both safer and more effective.

By adding natural, bio-identical hormones into your body, you can restore a good hormonal balance between estrogen and progesterone. Bio-identical hormones can be any of the steroid hormones, including estrogen, progesterone, or testosterone. However, many articles and blogs confuse people, making them think that natural or bio-identical hormones are the same as synthetic hormones. They are most definitely not. However, when I say bio-identical progesterone, I also mean natural progesterone and not synthetic progesterone. Using a natural or bio-identical progesterone is an important factor in correcting your underlying condition of estrogen dominance, resulting in loss of those unwanted pounds. By boosting your body's progesterone levels, you can offset the excess estrogen and create a proper hormonal balance that will allow your body to burn fat more efficiently.

So, why don't more physicians know about and prescribe bio-identical hormones?

The molecular structure of natural human hormones cannot be patented and neither can the identical molecular structure of bio-identical hormones. Without a patent, pharmaceutical companies cannot mass-produce, market, and sell them. No chance for big profits translates into no interest on the part of large pharmaceutical companies. Instead of selling the more natural products, pharmaceutical companies produce and patent synthetic hormones, which are patentable because they have a slightly different molecular structure from both natural human hormones and bio-identical hormones. These companies then spend millions of dollars marketing synthetic hormones to physicians (via office presentations, forums, and meetings) so that physicians will prescribe synthetic hormones rather than bio-identical ones. The companies make billions of dollars selling these synthetic hormones.

Despite numerous credible clinical trials and research studies that validate the safety and efficacy of bio-identical hormone therapies, many doctors remain unaware of their health benefits. This may be because many doctors feel that synthetic or prescription medicines in general are the best approach to addressing symptoms. However, many practitioners who study alternative medicine focus on healing the body, not just treating symptoms. Thus, they seek out the most effective natural methods for healing the body. This is my approach, of course. Others believe that many of the universities and establishments that publish information on bio-identical hormones don't have the budgets to educate and market to doctors, who are then slow to learn of their health benefits.

How Bio-identical Hormones Help in the Battle of the Bulge

By using bio-identical progesterone, you increase your progesterone levels to neutralize estrogen dominance. The proper balance between estrogen and progesterone will help your body efficiently metabolize food so that it is not stored as fat. Additionally, progesterone acts as a natural diuretic, reducing bloating and water weight. For those who are insulin resistant, you'll be glad to know that a better balance between progesterone and estrogen slows the rapid release of insulin, thereby decreasing fat storage in the body. There are also studies that show that bio-identical progesterone can reduce estrogen's ability to stimulate cell growth that can result in cancer, thereby providing additional protection against cancer. For younger, menstruating women, bio-identical progesterone is even used to help alleviate PMS symptoms.

How to Take Bio-identical Progesterone

Bio-identical progesterone can be taken as a cream, a pill, capsule, or as a suppository. However, topical creams have been shown to be the most effective way of taking it. If you take pills, you have to take a higher dosage because when the pill is digested, it must go through the liver to be metabolized, leaving much of the active ingredients to be excreted in the feces. So, only some of the active ingredient makes its way into the bloodstream to be used by the body. When you rub the cream form of it into your skin, it is absorbed directly into the bloodstream. Once it's in the bloodstream, the bio-identical progesterone can travel to the hormone receptor sites to be used by the body in the same manner human hormones would. As a result, a lower dosage is required when the bio-identical hormone topical cream is used.

The greatest success with bio-identical hormone replacement therapy occurs when you have the help of a trained healthcare provider who can provide an individual approach to address your hormonal imbalances. You should describe every symptom you experience while using bio-identical hormones, so that your healthcare provider can tweak the dosage of hormones until you reach a balanced hormonal state.

The provider should begin with laboratory tests of hormone levels (sometimes called "hormone panel") to understand your current hormone levels. The two most common types of hormone testing are saliva testing and blood testing. The correct prescription dosage, which is filled at a compounding pharmacy, will include customized bio-identical hormones based upon your hormonal levels. The doctor will then monitor you monthly to ensure that your symptoms are being alleviated. Follow-up hormone tests can also be conducted in four to six months to ensure hormonal balance is restored.

If you have difficulty finding a doctor who specializes in bio-identical hormones, check your local compounding pharmacy, as it may be able to recommend doctors with this specialization. Compounding pharmacies are where doctors in your area will call to fill your custom compound of bio-identical hormone prescriptions that are custom-prepared just for you based upon your individual needs. You can do a Google search to find local compounding pharmacies in your area or a doctor specializing in bio-identical hormone therapy.

Your healthcare provider should advise you on the most efficient method for taking progesterone. However, bio-identical progesterone cream is readily available without a prescription at most health food stores and health websites. Some women who opt to begin taking over-the-counter bio-identical hormones should be aware that some over-the-counter progesterone creams are better than others. Unfortunately, there is no regulatory body that oversees the production or standardization of natural health products. The closest standard for quality bio-identical hormone products is to ensure that it meets the U.S. Pharmacopoeia gold standard for quality. You can look for this distinction on the label. Additionally, Dr. John Lee, the leading authority and pioneer in the use of natural progesterone cream, offers a list of quality natural progesterone creams. The link to this list can be found here at www.johnleemd.com/store/resource_progesterone.html.

For more information on bio-identical hormone replacement therapy and ways to stay youthful and energetic, read these four excellent books: *Dr. John Lee's Hormone Balance Made Simple* by John R. Lee and Virginia Hopkins; *Ageless: The Naked Truth About Bio-identical Hormones* and *The Sexy Years: Discover the Hormone Connection: The Secret to Fabulous Sex, Great Health, and Vitality for Women and Men*, both by Suzanne Somers; and *The Miracle of Bio-Identical Hormones* by Michael E. Platt, M.D.

Supplements That Support Hormone Balance

When dealing with the most common form of hormonal imbalance, estrogen dominance, the most effective supplements are those that help eliminate excess estrogen from the body or metabolize estrogen so that more of the "good estrogen" is used by the body and more of the "bad estrogen" is eliminated from the body. The select group of supplements below has been proven to create hormone balance, resulting in weight loss and fewer mood swings, hot flashes, and other symptoms caused by hormonal imbalance. You should work with your healthcare provider to determine if any of these supplements would be beneficial to you.

Calcium D-Glucarate

Calcium D-glucarate is a common nutrient found in

many fruits and vegetables. This nutrient is believed to aid the body in the elimination of many harmful toxins and also lowers abnormally high levels of hormones, namely estrogen. Calcium D-glucarate inhibits the reabsorption of estrogen-mimicking toxins into the bloodstream, allowing them to be excreted out of the body. Women dealing with estrogen dominance can typically take 1,000 mg of calcium D-glucarate two times per day.

Dehydroepiandrosterone (DHEA)

Dehydroepiandrosterone (DHEA) is a steroid hormone produced by the body's adrenal glands. DHEA functions as a precursor to testosterone, the male sex hormone, and estrogen, the female sex hormone. In most people, DHEA production gradually declines with age, and it is believed that supplementing our bodies' falling levels of this hormone might help turn back the hands of time and boost the body's ability to burn fat. DHEA causes weight loss through a process called thermogenesis, which is the creation of heat at a cellular level. The more thermogenesis, the higher the metabolic rate, and the more fat burned. It is recommended that you take 100 mg of DHEA daily.

Diindolylmethane (DIM)

Diindolylmethane (DIM) is a phytonutrient, a plant compound similar to those found in cruciferous vegetables, such as broccoli, cabbage, Brussels sprouts, and cauliflower. Since it would be difficult to get enough of these vegetables through our diet daily (it would require eating two pounds of broccoli per day) to properly eliminate the bad estrogen, we can take a nutritional supplement known as DIM (diindolylmethane) to get the adequate amounts to restore hormonal balance and eliminate the symptoms of estrogen dominance. DIM eliminates excess estrogen by shifting the way estrogen is metabolized in the body. DIM allows for more of the "good estrogen" metabolites and elimination of the "bad estrogen" metabolites. DIM will not directly decrease the estrogen levels in the body, but rather will redirect how it is metabolized so that more of the "bad estrogen" metabolites are eliminated.

Consuming vegetables containing DIM or a DIM supplement can help prevent the development of certain cancers. DIM has also been proven to destroy and prevent the mutation of cancer cells. DIM is believed to help prevent breast and prostate cancer by promoting a balance of good vs. bad estrogen in the body.

Using a bio-identical progesterone cream in combination with DIM has been shown to even more effectively alleviate symptoms of estrogen dominance than just using the cream alone. One reason for this is that there's no ideal way to tell how much progesterone you're actually getting through the cream or how much your body is able to use, and taking the time to monitor symptoms and test for progesterone levels periodically makes the treatment a little bit slow. So, the use of DIM, along with a bio-identical progesterone cream, alleviates symptoms faster.

Many practitioners recommend taking about 200 to 300 mg of DIM per day (or about 100 to 150 mg twice per day). Since it is difficult to absorb, be sure it is in the form of a specialized complex to improve bioavailability. You don't want to take plain DIM without the bioavailable complex. There are very few reported side effects from taking supplemental DIM. However, some individuals have experienced headaches, upset stomach, and gas. If this occurs, be sure to take DIM with food and to reduce the dosage and slowly work your way up to the recommended dosage.

Tips for Preventing Weight Gain During Perimenopause and Menopause

In addition to exploring BHRT and taking nutritional supplements, eating right and staying physically active will help you maintain your ideal body weight during the perimenopause and menopause phases of life. All of the advice provided in the DEM System is especially helpful for women in perimenopause and menopause.

There are eight rules you can follow that will help you prevent weight gain during perimenopause/menopause. They are the following:

1. *Maintain healthy liver function* and regular bowel movements to eliminate excess estrogen from the body. Chapter 5 gave specific herbs and supplements that help cleanse and protect the liver.

2. *Avoid alcohol.* It spurs the production of harmful estrogen. In fact, even one glass of alcohol a day can raise estrogen levels.

3. *Minimize exposure to xenoestrogens.* These are environmental chemicals in pesticides, plastics, some cosmetics, and household cleaning products that can get into your bloodstream and increase estrogen levels.

4. *Eliminate sugar and starch from your diet.* Get sugar out of your diet if you want to lose body fat. By

sugar, I mean candy and sweets, of course, but really any starchy, processed foods that cause insulin spikes resulting in excess fat in the body. If you want to reduce fatigue and weight (fat) gain, try to have no more than two servings of starchy carbohydrates— such as potatoes and corn—per day and avoid sugary sweets altogether.

5. *Eat more fiber.* Fiber from whole grains, fruits, and vegetables helps to move estrogen out of the body, which helps prevent it from building up and creating a hormonal burden on your system.

6. *Eat lean proteins.* I discussed the value of lean protein earlier, but it really helps to offset the symptoms of perimenopause and menopause by helping maintain muscle mass, which burns more calories than fat. Whenever your body is not getting enough protein, you will begin to feel moody, emotional, anxious, and just plain tired. Good choices of protein are eggs, fish, lean beef, turkey, or chicken.

7. *Eat more detoxifying foods.* Add plenty of detoxifying foods to your diet, including broccoli, cauliflower, Brussels sprouts, kale, cabbage, beets, carrots, apples, ginger, onions, and celery. Eat at least five servings of fresh fruits and veggies per day. In particular, dark leafy green veggies, such as spinach, collards, and kale, are ideal. Regarding fruit, the brighter and deeper the color the better; great choices are oranges, blackberries, and apples.

8. *Get moving!* The unpleasant reality is that women begin to naturally lose muscle mass during middle

age. So not only are we gaining and storing fat, we're losing lean muscle mass as well. This is a double whammy. So you will want to begin some physical activity to help maintain lean muscle mass as you age to boost your metabolism. (See Chapter 12 for additional ideas on how to "get moving.")

At the time of this writing, I am in my forties and in perimenopause. I experienced many unpleasant symptoms of estrogen dominance, including acne, bloating, depression, hot flashes, heavy or painful periods, irregular periods, irritability, loss of muscle mass, mood swings, poor concentration, sleep disturbances, urinary incontinence, and, my least favorite, rapid unexplained weight gain. My rapid weight gain was actually alarming due to how healthy my lifestyle and eating habits were at the time.

I did my research and embraced bio-identical hormone replacement therapy and other nutritional supplements and herbs. Now, I have no problem with aging. I love being in my forties as long as I have a healthy, youthful, and energetic body. Balanced hormones bring joy, strength, and great physical and emotional health. I've learned from experience that a healthy woman is hormonally balanced.

If you are frustrated with belly fat, a pear-shaped body, or bloating and water retention, the use of bio-identical hormones and other key supplements can help you restore the hormone balance and metabolic function in the body. Fat distribution will normalize, and you will begin to see the weight melt away.

CHAPTER SIXTEEN

Don't Like to Exercise? Try SEXercise!

Sexercising routines not only help you get fit, they also help you get your sexy back. Keep in mind that men are very visual creatures, and having a little sex appeal will not only give you more confidence in your feminine self, but will also help you attract more men. There are four popular types of sexercises: pole dancing, belly dancing, Zumba, and striptease.

Pole Dancing

Although pole dancing is fast becoming a widely accepted fitness activity, there are still a lot of misconceptions about what it really is all about. Pole dancing allows many women to improve their confidence and self-esteem while becoming more fit and toned. If you get past the stigma that comes along with pole dancing, you'll find that it is a great way to build incredible strength while having loads of fun. The pole requires significant arm strength because most of the time you are using your arms to lift your entire body. There is a wide variety of exercises you can do on your pole to increase flexibility and muscle tone while performing sexy, strength-building dance moves.

Although pole dancing is associated with strippers,

there's no nudity at a pole-dancing class nor are there men gawking at you during the class session. You will find women of all ages and sizes prancing around the pole, flying in the air, and spinning forward and backward, with pauses for little playful teases. Throughout the class session, students learn different pole exercise moves and eventually work their way up to performing a complete routine. Many take their newfound skills and offer their boyfriend or husband a special treat. Some join to get fit, embrace their sexuality, or simply to gain more self-confidence. Whatever the reason they join, they typically leave feeling sexy, sensual, and confident about their bodies. Pole-dancing fitness can liberate your sensuality and give you confidence in showing off your new feminine body.

Belly Dancing

Belly dancing is not only fun but is also a great form of exercise. It tones the arms, strengthens and tightens the abs and obliques, and improves flexibility. It can burn as many calories as jogging, swimming, or riding a bike but is less strenuous on the body than weight lifting and more entertaining than sitting on a bike at the gym.

Belly dancing is a very different form of exercise than what you may be used to, as it is a beautiful and sensual dance form. What makes belly dancing unique is that it is a cultural experience; you learn about its Middle Eastern origins while burning fat, improving flexibility and posture, and enhancing your sexuality and femininity. Belly dancing is great for women who want sexy abs, as it's a perfect workout for your midsection, waist, and core. Belly dancing adds a whole different dimension to your fitness experience.

Zumba

Zumba is a type of fitness class that has garnered quite a bit of attention recently. A great way to firm, tone, and sweat while doing a lively, upbeat Latin dance, Zumba incorporates aerobic interval training with Latin-style dance movements to provide a refreshing change from traditional aerobics routines. Many are enamored with Zumba's many benefits for burning fat, toning muscles, and having fun. Zumba classes, which usually last about an hour, can burn up to 500 calories and really rev up your metabolism. It's a fun workout that is more of a good time than an exercise class.

The dance moves are easy to learn. Instructors teach the basic routines and then add more intricate dance moves. The movements used in Zumba—such as salsa, merengue, cha-cha, mambo, and Zumba shuffle steps—all help to tone muscles. Zumba feels more like an evening at a Latin dance club than an exercise routine and is growing in popularity each day.

Striptease

Striptease is more of a seductive dance routine, typically performed in stilettos. When I attended striptease class, the dips and gyrating leg movements really helped to tone up my thighs and legs. Both striptease and pole-dance classes are great ways to embrace your sexuality and simply look and feel sexy and desirable. There are also workout videos, like Flirty Girl Fitness DVDs, if you want to work out at home as opposed to going to a dance studio.

Striptease is an exercise routine that you may prefer to practice in the privacy of your own home. This will allow you to let go of your inhibitions. The more you practice, the more you'll get comfortable freeing your sensual self. The good news is that you really begin to work your muscles by gyrating and bending to the music of your choice. Once you get comfortable with your striptease routine, you may want to show it to your significant other. I'm sure he will enjoy your lean and toned body, along with your sensuality. When you get confident in your body, your movements will be beautiful and sensual, and you'll walk around the room with a wonderful, sexual presence that you and your mate will both appreciate.

CHAPTER SEVENTEEN

Why Black Women Gain More Weight Than Other Women

The statistics are widely published. The National Center for Health Statistics reports that more than one half (54.3 percent) of Americans are obese, with black women comprising the most overweight segment of the U.S. population, followed by Hispanic women. The statistics indicate that 78 percent of us are overweight—that's nearly four out of five black women—and 54 percent of us are obese. African-American women are suffering from obesity at an alarmingly disproportionate rate compared to women of other races.

As I've said earlier, being overweight or obese is not always a matter of eating too much or not exercising, but this gets even more complicated for black women. There are a variety of reasons that black women are overweight or obese. I will discuss five of them in this section.

Black Woman Have a Slower Metabolism

Genetically, African-American women tend to have a slower metabolism, according to research published in the *American Journal of Clinical Nutrition*. A University of Pennsylvania Medical Center study found that black women have "a biological disadvantage" that makes it more difficult to lose weight. Researchers have found that even at rest, overweight black women burn nearly 100 fewer calories daily compared to their overweight white peers. While this news may seem like gloom and doom for black women who want to lose weight, know that it is a challenge that can be overcome. The healthy eating and lifestyle strategies described in this book, specifically the ways to speed up your metabolism (see Chapter 7), will help you burn more calories.

Black Women Are More Prone to Insulin Resistance, Which Causes Excess Fat Storage in the Body

Black women, even if their weight is normal, may be at increased risk for insulin resistance, a condition linked to diabetes and high blood pressure, according to research by Wake Forest University School of Medicine. Insulin resistance means the body can't effectively use the hormone insulin to process glucose, forcing the pancreas to produce more insulin, and elevated insulin levels lead to excess fat storage in the body. Almost half of lean black women had insulin resistance, which was double the rate in both Hispanic and Caucasian women. The study showed that 47 percent of black women of normal weight had insulin resistance compared to less than 20 percent of the Hispanic or Caucasian women.

The researchers looked at how obesity relates to insulin resistance in Black, Caucasian, and Hispanic women as a part of the Insulin Resistance Atherosclerosis Study (IRAS). The research suggested that race, in addition to obesity, is an important contributor to the development of insulin resistance and type-2 diabetes. This means that black women, even when lean, have a higher risk of developing insulin resistance, which leads to excess fat storage in the body if not properly treated.

Blacks May Have a "Thrifty Gene" Causing Them to Eat More

There is a so-called thrifty gene that helps the body to function on a minimal amount of food. Some researchers believe that African Americans inherited such a gene from their African ancestors. Years ago, this gene enabled Africans, during "feast and famine" cycles, to use food energy more efficiently when food was scarce. People possessing the thrifty gene, which includes African Americans, have a problem in that their built-in appetite suppressant (leptin) doesn't seem to work. Apparently, this gene has lingered from former times when food was not readily available. These people became "leptin resistant," which means their bodies ignore hormonal messages to stop eating and to stop storing fat. This happened because when food was not readily available, their bodies adapted to hold on to fat stores so they could remain alive in those lean times.

Black Women Can Carry More Weight and Still Be Healthy

According to a report by *Reuters Health*, in a 2011 study conducted by Peter T. Katzmarzyk, associate executive director for Population Science, and his colleagues at the Pennington Biomedical Research Center, black women can carry more weight than white women and still be considered healthy. Katzmarzyk's group calculated the body mass indexes (BMIs) and measured the waist circumferences of over six thousand men and women of all races to look for the threshold at which weight becomes significantly associated with disease. According to the National Institutes of Health's Clinical Guidelines on the Identification, Evaluation, and Treatment of Overweight and Obesity in Adults, a BMI of 30 or higher is linked to more cases of high cholesterol, diabetes, and high blood pressure. But Katzmarzyk found that the cutoff does not seem to hold true for black women. While there was no racial difference for men, Katzmarzyk showed that, for black women, the risk didn't increase until they reached a BMI of 33. Dr. Katzmarzyk thought a possible reason for the contrast might be the difference in the way body fat is distributed in women among the races. So, being skinny (with a low BMI) does not indicate a healthy body, but rather, getting healthy should be the focus of our weight loss efforts. Getting a healthy body is key to having a beautiful body.

Many Black Women Are Prone to Emotional Eating

Many black women have had to become heads of households, hold down multiple jobs, and raise kids alone. Eating may become a way to deal with the stress and disappointments of life. But unfortunately, weight gain leads to chronic illness. Mortality rates for black women are higher than that for any other racial/ethnic group in nearly every major cause of death, including heart disease, lung cancer, and breast cancer. We are the lifegivers, the caregivers, and think it is our job to take care of everyone but ourselves. However, self-love demands that we take care of ourselves first, so we can give to others from our abundance. We must become accountable to ourselves.

Many black women feel that being thick or "phat"—"pretty hot and tempting"—is cute or sexy. However, we must know when *phat* is actually *fat* that needs to be burned away to reveal a slim, healthier body. To my sistas, it's time to lose weight and save your life; you've got a lot of living left to do!

CHAPTER EIGHTEEN

Motivation for a New Body and a New You

I watched Terrell "Zero Body Fat" Owens on the sideline emphatically say, "I love me some me!" He said it with so much passion and conviction that I knew he meant it! So that got me to wondering, how I can actually "love me some me." I believe it has to start with improving the relationship I have with myself.

If you love yourself and have confidence in who you are, you'll begin to send a signal to others that you have value and deserve respect. Loving yourself first sends a clear message that you are to be recognized, celebrated, appreciated, and loved. Sometimes our sense of self-worth or self-esteem is shaped by the people in our inner circle. Some of us have family members and friends ruining our self-esteem every day. Even if they are your flesh and blood, try to remove yourself from their presence as much as possible. Hurtful words negate any progress toward self-worth and self-love.

Let Self-Love Heal Your Mind, Body, and Spirit

Self-love is key to maintaining your healthy, ideal weight. The body has a natural ability to create and maintain the perfect weight for you as long as you are aligned with your true self. For in your true self is everything that is good and perfect about you. By getting back to the truth of who you really are, the real you, you will get to a place where all your problems with weight begin to disappear. Only the power of love can help you find your true self. You have to understand love, a power that is greater than your own. In fact, it's greater than any addiction or eating disorder that you may have. Learning to love will allow you to overcome the power of hate because the truth is that unhealthy eating is an act of self-hate.

The power of love is perfect, healthy, all-knowing, self-healing, and abundant. In contrast, the power of fear is destructive, chaotic, and lacking. It expresses itself as an impostor, causing you to act against your true nature. You have to grow spiritually to understand the power of both love and fear. Both of them are always present and active, but one wishes you health and happiness and the other wishes you death and destruction.

Self-love is essential to survival. There is no successful, authentic relationship with others without self-love. We cannot nurture others from a dry well. It is not selfish or self-indulgent. We have to take care of our needs first so we can give to others from our abundance. You will have to love yourself and love your body. Whether you feel fat or overweight, you have to love your body now, unconditionally. If you can't love your body now, then you can't truly love yourself unconditionally. If you can't love your body because you don't like the way it looks, then know that the reasons you became overweight were not all your fault. But now that you have new knowledge about healthy eating, it's time to forgive yourself and others so you can let go of your old body and move toward your slimmer, healthier body.

When you understand the power of love, you can actually love food and make it your friend rather than your enemy. Food nourishes and sustains you; it cements your relationships with family members and friends. Food is meant to be eaten and enjoyed...but in moderation. You are not a slave to food. You eat when you are hungry, but you can leave food alone if you are not.

The only way to attain a healthy relationship with food is to learn to love it and ensure that the food you put into your body loves you back: it fuels you, nourishes you, and supports your optimal health and vitality. A candy bar does not love you—it's full of sugar and processed chemicals that harm your body. The people who made it don't love you, either—they are just trying to make money by selling you a product. Chemicals and processed foods lead to poor health, sickness, food allergies, ailments, and other diseases, none of which I would classify as "loving" conditions. So, if you are in a place where you still desire candy, that just means that you're still growing spiritually and have not reached your highest, true self. When you do, you won't desire foods that are harmful to your health.

Foods that love you are those that contribute to your health and wellness, such as fruits, nuts and seeds, and vegetables. These healthy, natural foods make your body stronger and able to fight illness and disease and have beauty and vibrancy. Natural, healthy foods make your body strong, fight illness, restore your body, produce beautiful skin, revitalize your mind, give you energy, slow the aging process, and will taste so much better than you can imagine once your taste buds have been reprogrammed. You have to be deliberate about finding healthy foods because unhealthy foods are readily available and easily accessible. But in some instances, I bet you have driven right by the farmers' market or health food store. It's time to make a stop there and begin to change your life.

Don't stress about trying to stop eating unhealthy foods at the beginning of your journey. It is a process that involves breaking your addictions to the many unhealthy foods you eat and think you "love" today. Just be aware of exactly what you're eating and know that there will come a day when you will no longer love foods that don't love you.

For me, I overcame my addiction to sugar, sweets, and junk food over time by taking gradual steps. Instead of eating regular chocolate chip cookies with refined white sugar, I began to eat sugar-free cookies that contained artificial sweeteners. Although they were not very healthy, either due to the white flour, trans fats, and artificial sweeteners they contained, they did help me break my addiction to white refined sugar. However, a few months later, once I learned about the dangers of artificial sweeteners and trans fats, I stopped eating sugar-free cookies as well. You will find the right approach for how you transition to more healthy foods that is right for you.

For some people, overeating is a way to cope with painful feelings and emotions. Being overweight and overeating tends to be a relationship issue. You hide behind your weight issues. You have built a wall around yourself, making you unavailable to new friendships and love.

To begin loving your body and your true self, post the following affirmative statements on a note card and read them every day before you leave for work:

1. I will have a loving relationship with food. I know that food is a gift from God that I am grateful for because it nourishes my body.

2. I am thankful for my body and look forward to a slimmer, healthier body as I become more enlightened about healthy eating.

3. I will not be afraid to get on the scale because the number that I weigh isn't as important as the overall healthiness of my body. A healthy body is a beautiful body.

4. I will not be ashamed of my body, for it is just the house for my spiritual and mental self; it does not define my true self.

5. I will forgive myself and other people. No more arguing and fighting, only letting go of stresses, failures, and disappointments.

To take your first step toward attaining self-love, you need to evaluate your self-image. Your self-image comes from and is reflected by the thoughts and feelings you have formed and integrated throughout your lifetime. A poor self-image leads to unsuccessful, self-defeating behavior that negatively affects your relationships and overall health. If you lack self-love and treat yourself as unimportant, others will see you as unimportant as well. If you feel yourself unworthy of the time and effort required to lose weight, then it is unlikely that you will grow healthier and happier.

If you are constantly worrying about your weight and always have negative thoughts and feelings that make you unhappy with yourself, it's time to break out of that cycle. If you catch yourself saying negative things to yourself or about yourself, stop and replace those thoughts with positive ones. Say the positive thought out loud. As an example, if you're thinking "my stomach is so huge," stop yourself and say, "I am excited about how beautiful my body will be when I lose a few pounds." The more you practice this method, the more you begin to change your inner life.

Don't allow negative thoughts to linger in your mind. Be diligent about pushing negative thoughts out of your mind and instantly replacing them with thoughts that are encouraging or positive. Don't be wishy-washy about your positive statements, either. Don't say, "I hope to lose weight" or "I'm trying to lose thirty pounds." Instead, say, "I *will* lose thirty pounds. I *will* have a slimmer body that makes me feel sexy." You're not planning, wishing, or hoping—you are doing it! Thoughts and feelings have power that can help or hurt you. Changing your thoughts changes your life.

Beware of Emotional Eating

Do you eat when you're sad, hurt, or lonely? Emotional eating almost always leads to inappropriate eating. Without realizing it, you may be caught in a vicious cycle of "living to eat," not "eating to live." Just the same as a drug or alcohol addict, you have to make sure that you don't use food to escape your problems. Food should be seen for what it is: fuel for the body to give it energy and vitality.

An important way to address emotional eating is to learn the difference between emotional hunger and physical hunger. This is absolutely key. Sometimes our relationship with food is an emotional one rather than a physical one. Sometimes we eat to fill an emotional gap or some other negative emotion. But no food, cracker, cake, ice cream, or pie can satisfy emotional hunger.

Emotional hunger comes on suddenly—*I must eat something now*. But you rarely feel satisfied or full, and so you just keep eating and eating until the entire bag of chips or pint of ice cream is gone. If the hunger comes on after an argument or a negative emotion, then it is emotional hunger. You need to learn to deal with the emotions head on.

Physical hunger comes about gradually about every three to four hours. Watch the clock. If you ate a meal and were full one hour ago and then feel a sudden need to eat something, it's probably emotional hunger.

Dealing with your emotional issues will help you improve your relationship with food. To deal with your emotions, you must come to understand that the bad things that have happened in your life have probably been floating around in your mind for years, and because you try to suppress these feelings, as most of us do, they have never been properly processed.

When we dwell on the sad events of our lives, they get etched in our minds, stuck in our bodies, weighing us down emotionally. We must process these experiences and let them go. If we don't, the negative emotions become toxic to our emotional and physical body. Sad or painful experiences are meant to teach us lessons we needed to learn so that we could grow and mature as a person—they are not meant to linger for years and years.

Just as we can get rid of toxic wastes in the body, we can get rid of toxic emotions. Instead of eating to distract ourselves from bad feelings, we need to process and eliminate them—just like the body does with food: it takes the nutrients it needs and expels the rest.

Part of expelling negative emotions involves forgiveness, of yourself and others. Authors Stephen Kendrick and Alex Kendrick discuss forgiveness in their book *The Love Dare* in the following terms:

> "Forgiveness doesn't clear anyone of blame. It doesn't clear their record with God. It just clears YOU of having to worry about how to punish them. When you forgive another person, you're not turning them loose, but turning them over to God, who can be counted on to deal with them His way. You're saving yourself the trouble of arguing and fighting. It's not about winning and losing anymore. It's about LETTING GO!"

Tips for Staying Motivated

In order to ensure success on the DEM System, you may want to follow these tips to stay motivated and committed.

Have an attitude of self-forgiveness. You must forgive yourself for the poor and destructive eating habits you've had for so many years. You are like many others in that you have been on the Standard American Diet. However, you cannot move forward in losing weight permanently and restoring optimal health without self-forgiveness.

290

Additionally, you must also forgive friends, family, and others who have fed you an unhealthy diet over the years, as they probably didn't know any better and did the best they could with what they knew at the time. You will sometimes make bad decisions in terms of what you eat. We all lose control and make bad food choices, but it is important to know that one bad decision doesn't have to turn into two or three. The key to weight loss and staying confident is to decrease the number of bad decisions you make on a daily basis.

Make your health a priority. You must begin thinking differently. First, decide that your health is one of the top priorities in your life. Know that your body is naturally thin. If you prepare your mind and absorb the knowledge offered to you in this book, you will have all the power you need to become your best self and transform your life in every way. Even if you are a busy mom or high-powered career executive, know that today begins the journey toward your most amazing, beautiful self. It is time to treat your body as the greatest gift that you have. It is time to shine as the person you were always meant to be. When you have a healthy and positive energy in life, amazing things like love, joy, success, and wealth come your way. Every interaction at work, church, home, or in the streets can be simply magnetic. Get healthy, lose weight, and watch your entire life begin to change for the better.

List ten reasons why you want to lose weight. Give serious thought to this list and ensure that each reason reflects your true goals and desires and that the list is meaningful to you. The reasons should be highly personal and not meant to please anyone but yourself. These become your personal motivators. Read them every day. You may even want to post them at work or carry them in your purse or wallet on an index card. You will need to remind yourself of these motivators to keep yourself focused.

Visualize your goals. What will your life look like when you're thinner and healthier? Visualize your perfect body and get comfortable with the idea it will be yours by the end of this program. Everything in life is made up of energy, including your thoughts. Positive thoughts attract positive energy. Negative thoughts attract negative energy. What you think is what you become. If you think of yourself as slim and healthy, you will begin to move in the direction of being thin and healthy. Don't think about being overweight, think about being thin. See yourself as having an attractive, sexy, energetic body. Allow your thoughts to work with your efforts of changing your eating habits so that you accelerate your progress, having everything in your life working with you, not against you.

Engage in positive self-talk. Thoughts and feelings turn into actions, and actions into reality. Remember, you are beginning a new chapter in your life. Let me encourage you right now to get started with your journey. Many ask, "How do I start?" or "How do I get there?" Well, it begins with positive self-talk. You want to stop thinking and saying negative things about yourself. You are not fat, lazy, ugly, or sick. Your true self is naturally thin, beautiful, and healthy. If you have negative thoughts about yourself, you'll attract negative people and outcomes in your life. If you say that you can never lose weight, you're exactly right: you won't. If you say you can, your subconscious mind believes that and begins to move your actions in the direction of losing weight.

Don't get obsessed with weighing yourself every day. Don't let your bathroom scale ruin your motivation. Frequent weighing can be confusing, so focus on how your clothes look and feel on your body. Scales are reliable over the long haul but give you inaccurate day-to-day reads. Weight fluctuations can be caused by hormonal changes or fluid shifts and can lead to unnecessary disappointment. It can show gains or losses that are not there because most basic scales can't tell the difference between fat, muscle, and water weight. Your weight also fluctuates by several pounds throughout the day, and weighing yourself too much will only be confusing and discouraging. Plan on weighing yourself only once a week at the same time of day and wearing the same clothing or no clothing (naked is best). Focus on losing inches and on how you begin to feel, not just on pounds. With this program, you will be doing great things for your body and health. The number on the scale will take care of itself. Be happy with losing one to two pounds per week. If you do this for two months, you will be down by sixteen pounds.

Focus on losing body fat, not just weight. It's fine to have a weight goal to use as a guideline, but also focus on measuring and monitoring overall body fat as a percentage of overall weight. This will ensure that you lose fat, not muscle. Healthful body-fat percentages for men begin at about 8 percent; 22 percent for women. These percentages will keep you in a healthy, safe zone that will lower your risk for disease. If you only have a regular scale and want to get detailed body-fat measurements, you can invest in a home body-fat scale. A decent one will cost you about $100 to $200. I own one by Tanita that measures weight, body-fat percentages, and muscle mass and helps me get the best picture of my overall health. Once you begin to measure your body fat, you will be able to track the loss of the thing you really want to lose.

Take a picture! Looking at before and after pictures of your new body can be highly motivating. Of course, you'll be getting comments and compliments from friends, family, and coworkers, but nothing is as special as seeing with your very own eyes your new healthy, beautiful body. Health is important, but I understand your need to improve your physical appearance as well. So get out the camera and take photos as you progress along your weight-loss journey.

The reason some people look and feel better than others is that they work at it. Why do you think celebrities look so fabulous despite their age? It's because they are constantly thinking about their appearance. Their livelihood depends upon how good they look. However, anyone can commit to looking fabulous all the time. You can make the choice to eat whole, healthy foods instead of junk foods, stay active, drink lots of water, and get plenty of rest and relaxation. Yes, it takes more work and discipline to look great as you age, but you will reap the benefits of being your best, beautiful self.

Conclusion

Congratulations on taking control of your health by caring for your body and feeding it what it needs to be slim, healthy, and vibrant! You will reap the rewards now and continue to enjoy a lifestyle of optimal health and happiness. By participating in the DEM System, you will enjoy healthy foods, support your body with nutritional supplements, cleanse your body through various detox methods, and stay physically active. Be sure to always make time to nourish your inner spirit and soul by giving your body the rest and relaxation it needs to stay strong and healthy. You have given yourself a wonderful gift of optimal health and wellness.

The following are your marching orders for the rest of your long and healthy life:

- Detox weekly to eliminate toxins that cause fat cells.
- Eat "clean and balanced" foods and eliminate sugary foods.
- Take the necessary nutritional supplements.
- Get physically active and keep moving daily.
- Drink lots of water.
- Get as much sleep, rest, and relaxation as you need!

My own commitment to this lifestyle is unwavering due to the amazing results that I have experienced. My forty-plus-year-old body always feels wonderful—youthful and energetic. I never worry about putting on excess weight or returning to the poor state of health that I had in my twenties and thirties. I do not have some special gene that keeps me slim. I could gain excess weight like the next person without this system of healthy living. This lifestyle has benefited my clients, who have had some great successes as well. I know that you can—and will—reach your ideal weight and greatest health!

Remember that you have the power to change your life, and now with the information in this book, you have the tools to turn your dreams into reality. Every day is the beginning of the rest of your life. You are in control of what happens today. Start dreaming about a sexy, beautiful body and watch it become reality. You have power over your body and your life, so live it with passion because you only get one!

In closing, I wanted to leave you with my 10 Commandments for Looking Young and Feeling Great, which I always share at the end of my teleseminars.

1. *Thou shalt love thyself.* Self-love is essential to survival. There is no successful, authentic relationship with others without self-love. We cannot water the land from a dry well. Self-love is not selfish or self-indulgent. We have to take care of our needs first so we can give to others from abundance.

2. *Thou shalt take responsibility for thine own health and well-being.* If you want to be healthy, have more energy, and feel great, you must take the time to learn what is involved and apply it to your own life. You

have to watch what goes into your mouth, how much exercise or physical activity you get, and what thoughts you're thinking throughout the day.

3. *Thou shalt sleep.* Sleep and rest is the body's way of recharging the system. Sleep is the easiest, yet most underrated activity for healing the body. Lack of sleep definitely saps your glow and instantly ages you, giving you puffy red eyes with dark circles under them.

4. *Thou shalt detoxify and cleanse the body.* Detoxifying the body means ridding the body of poisons and toxins so that you can speed up weight loss and restore great health. A clean body is a beautiful body!

5. *Thou shalt remember that a healthy body is a sexy body.* Real women's bodies look beautiful! It's about getting healthy and having style and confidence and wearing clothes that match your body type.

6. *Thou shalt eat more healthy, natural, whole foods.* Healthy eating can turn back the hands of time and return the body to a more youthful state. When you eat natural foods, you simply look and feel better. You keep the body clean at the cellular level and look radiant despite your age. Eating healthy should be part of your "beauty regimen."

7. *Thou shalt embrace healthy aging.* The goal is not to stop the aging process but to embrace it. Healthy aging is staying healthy as you age, which is looking and feeling great despite your age.

8. *Thou shalt commit to a lifestyle change.* Losing weight permanently requires a commitment to changes...in

your thinking, your lifestyle, your mindset. It requires gaining knowledge and making permanent changes in your life for the better!

9. *Thou shalt embrace the journey.* This is a journey that will change your life; it's not a diet but a lifestyle! Be kind and supportive to yourself. Learn to applaud yourself for the smallest accomplishment. And when you slip up sometimes, know that it is okay; it is called being human.

10. *Thou shalt live, love, and laugh.* Laughter is still good for the soul. Live your life with passion! Never give up on your dreams! And most importantly...love! Remember that love never fails!

Now that you have experienced the power of the DEM System, be sure to share your success story with others and help them to reclaim their health and vitality.

APPENDIX A

Seven-Day Meal Plan and Recipes

This seven-day meal plan, with recipes, provides a sample meal plan to help you get started on the three-week Detox Phase of the DEM System. This meal plan and recipes will help you focus on foods that cleanse and detoxify the body while you re-program your taste buds to crave natural, healthy foods that help you get slim and healthy!

Seven-Day Meal Plan:

Day One
Breakfast:
- Almond Butter Oatmeal

Lunch:
- Quinoa Pilaf

Dinner:
- Walnut and Apple Spinach Salad

Snacks:
- 1 Apple
- Lightly Salted Popcorn

Day Two

Breakfast:

- Cottage Cheese and Berries

Lunch:

- Navy Bean and Barley Soup
- Whole-Grain Crackers

Dinner:

- Spinach Salad with Vinaigrette Dressing

Snacks:

- 1 cup Strawberries
- Unsweetened Peanut Butter with Celery

Day Three

Breakfast:

- Granola Berry Parfait

Lunch:

- Black Bean Quinoa Salad

Dinner:

- Black-Eyed Peas and Veggie-Stuffed Peppers

Snacks:

- 1 cup Blueberries
- 1 plain Yogurt with Berries

Day Four

Breakfast:

- Whole-Grain Hot or Cold Cereal (Brands by Ezekiel 4:9 or Bob's Red Mill's are great options)
- Unsweetened Almond Milk

Lunch:

- Sautéed Tomatoes and Spinach

Dinner:

- Green Leafy Stir Fry

Snacks:

- 1 Orange
- 1 Hard-Boiled Egg

Day Five

Breakfast:

- Basic Healthy Oatmeal with Toppings

Lunch:

- Basic Caesar Salad

Dinner:

- Marinated Veggie Stir-fry with Brown Rice

Snacks:

- 1 Apple
- Lightly Salted Popcorn

Day Six

Breakfast:

- Cinnamon Granola

Lunch:

- Cucumber Tomato Salad

Dinner:

- Braised Tofu
- Sweet Potato Fries
- Side Salad

Snacks:

- 1 cup Raspberries
- 1 cup Carrots

Day Seven

Breakfast:

- Whole-Grain Hot or Cold Cereal (Brands by Ezekiel 4:9 or Bob's Red Mill's are great options)
- Unsweetened Almond Milk

Lunch:

- Collard Green Stew with Black-Eyed Peas

Dinner:

- Marinated Veggie Stir-fry with Brown Rice

Snacks:

- 1 Pear
- Unsweetened Almond Butter with Celery

Recipes For the Seven-Day Meal Plan

Almond Butter Oatmeal

Ingredients:

- 1 cup cooked oats
  (cooked in unsweetened almond milk)
- 2 tablespoons almond butter
- 1 teaspoon cinnamon
- 1 tablespoon honey

Directions:

1. Make sure the oats are warm so everything melts properly.
2. Combine all ingredients in a bowl and mix until well combined.

Quinoa Pilaf

Ingredients:

- 1 cup uncooked quinoa
- 1 cup uncooked red lentils
- 1 medium red bell pepper, chopped
- ¼ cup raisins
- 2 tablespoons of extra-virgin olive oil
- ¼ cup orange juice (fresh squeezed is best)
- ¼ cup apple cider vinegar
- ½ cup roasted cashews, chopped
- 2 cloves garlic, peeled and chopped finely
- 2 tablespoons tamari

- 1 teaspoon caraway seeds
- ½ teaspoon red pepper flakes
- ½ teaspoon sea salt to taste

Directions:

1. Rinse and cook quinoa in 2 quarts of water for 10 minutes; drain and let cool.
2. Combine all other ingredients in a large bowl EXCEPT for the cashews.
3. Add cashews when ready to eat.

Walnut and Apple Spinach Salad

Ingredients:

- 6 ounces of baby spinach, washed
- ½ cup walnuts
- 2 large green apples, cut into thin slices
- 2 tablespoons golden raisins
- 3 tablespoons chopped red onion
- 2 tablespoons extra-virgin olive oil
- 2 tablespoons white wine vinegar
- 1 tablespoon honey
- ½ teaspoon sea salt
- ½ teaspoon ground black pepper
- 3 ounces reduced-fat crumbled goat cheese

Directions:

1. Toast the walnuts in a large, nonstick skillet over medium heat, stirring every 3 to 4 minutes. Let cool on a plate.

2. Whisk the oil, vinegar, honey, sea salt, and pepper in salad bowl.

3. Stir in the onions, apples, and raisins and then add the spinach and toss to coat evenly.

4. Sprinkle on walnuts and goat cheese before serving.

Cottage Cheese and Berries

Ingredients:

- ½ cup low-fat or nonfat cottage cheese
- ¼ cup fresh blueberries
- ¼ cup fresh strawberries, chopped
- ¼ cup walnuts

Directions:

1. Combine and mix all the ingredients in one bowl and serve.

Navy Bean and Barley Soup

Ingredients:

- 2 cans navy beans
- 3 large carrots
- 1 pound package of frozen peas
- 4 stalks celery
- 8 cups veggie stock
- 4 teaspoons fresh oregano
- ½ cup cooked barley

Directions:

1. Place veggie stock, herbs, celery, carrots, and frozen peas into the pot and bring to a boil.

2. Once the veggies are cooked (soft to touch), add in the navy beans and cook long enough to warm the beans.

3. Put the barley into a bowl and top with soup. Add sea salt to taste.

Spinach Salad with Vinaigrette Dressing

Ingredients:

- 6 cups loosely packed baby spinach

- 1 cup strawberries (without stem)

- ¼ cup toasted pumpkin seeds

- Vinaigrette Dressing:

> ¼ cup extra-virgin olive oil
>
> 2 tablespoons red wine vinegar
>
> 1 teaspoon Dijon mustard
>
> 1 teaspoon agave
>
> Pinch of sea salt

Directions:

1. Place spinach and ½ cup strawberries in large bowl.

2. In small bowl, whisk together vinaigrette dressing ingredients.

3. Pour over salad and toss to coat evenly.

4. Top with remaining seeds and strawberries.

Granola Berry Parfait

Ingredients:

- ½ cup raspberries
- ½ cup blueberries
- 1 banana sliced
- 1 ½ cups granola
- 1 container of soy yogurt

Directions:

1. Layer the banana, blueberries, raspberries, yogurt, and granola in 2 tall glasses
2. Serve immediately.

Black Bean Quinoa Salad

Ingredients:

- 1 can black beans
- 2 cups cooked quinoa
- 1 mango, peeled and cut into small pieces
- 1 red bell pepper, diced into small pieces
- 1 cup green onions, chopped
- 1 cup fresh parsley, chopped
- 2 tablespoons red wine vinegar
- 2 tablespoons grapeseed oil
- ¼ teaspoon sea salt

Directions:

1. Combine the red bell pepper, green onions, mango, and parsley in a mixing bowl.

2. Add the red wine vinegar, grapeseed oil, and sea salt and stir them up.

3. Add the quinoa and stir all of the ingredients. Gently fold in the black beans.

4. Serve at room temperature or chill beforehand.

Black-Eyed Peas and Veggie Stuffed Pepper

Ingredients:

- 2 cans black-eyed peas, drained and rinsed
- 1 can diced tomatoes
- 1 cup diced carrots
- 2 jalapenos, sliced finely
- 1 medium yellow onion, finely chopped
- 4 large bell peppers, cut in half lengthwise
- 2 tablespoons extra-virgin olive oil
- 4 garlic cloves, chopped finely
- 2 dried bay leaves
- 1 teaspoon dried oregano
- 1 teaspoon dried basil
- 2 teaspoons paprika
- 3 sprigs of fresh thyme
- 1 teaspoon sea salt
- ¼ cup fresh parsley, chopped

Directions:

1. Heat oven to 350° F and spray 9 x 13 pan with olive oil.

2. Bring a large pot of water to a boil and put the bell peppers in the water to boil for 5 minutes; let them drain and then cool.

3. Over medium-high heat, warm the oil in large skillet and sauté the onions, carrots, and jalapeno peppers for 5 minutes. Add the garlic and sauté an additional 5 minutes.

4. Add the other herbs, spices, and sea salt and sauté for another minute.

5. Add the tomatoes and peas and stir and cover for 10 minutes and then mix in the parsley.

6. Remove the bay leaves and thyme sprigs and add a half cup of the veggie mixture into each pepper half.

7. Place the pepper halves into the 9 x 13–pan and bake for 25 minutes.

Sautéed Tomatoes and Spinach

Ingredients:

- 2 plum tomatoes, seeded and diced
- 1 bunch of spinach (6 cups loosely packed)
- 2 tablespoons grapeseed oil
- 1 small onion, chopped finely
- 3 garlic cloves, minced
- 2 teaspoons fresh ginger
- ½ teaspoon sea salt
- ½ lemon

Directions:

1. Heat a large skillet over medium-high heat and sauté the onions in the oil for 2 minutes.

2. Add in the ginger, garlic, and sea salt and sauté for another 30 seconds.

3. Add in the tomatoes and sauté for about 2 minutes.

4. Add in the spinach and cook until the spinach is wilted; add splashes of water so that the spinach doesn't burn.

5. Sprinkle in lemon juice and serve.

Green Leafy Stir-fry

Ingredients:

- 1 pound of dark green, leafy veggies (such as collards, kale, spinach, mustard greens, dandelion greens, etc.)

- 2 tablespoons peanut oil

- 3 cloves of garlic, chopped finely

- ½-inch cube of ginger, peeled and grated

- 1 tablespoon cooking sherry

- 2 teaspoons soy sauce

- 1 teaspoon sesame oil

- Pinch of raw sugar

Directions:

1. Slice greens into 1-inch wide sections and wash and dry greens.

2. In a large nonstick skillet, heat the peanut oil over medium-high heat and add in the garlic and ginger.

3. Cook, stirring constantly, for a few minutes or until stems begin to soften.

Basic Healthy Oatmeal

Ingredients:

- 1 ¼ cups water

- 1 cup rolled oats

- ⅓ to ½ teaspoon stevia powder (sweeten to taste)

- ¹⁄₁₆ teaspoon sea salt (optional)

- Toppings (unsweetened almond milk, berries, almonds, raisins, cinnamon)

Directions:

1. Place water and salt in a medium pan and bring to a boil and stir in oats.

2. Reduce heat to medium and cook for an additional 5 minutes, stirring as needed.

3. Remove from heat, cover, and let sit for 4 to 5 minutes.

4. Sprinkle with stevia and add in any of the toppings above.

Basic Caesar Salad

Ingredients:

- 1 head of romaine lettuce torn into bite-size pieces

- 1 tablespoon fresh lemon juice
- 1 teaspoon apple cider vinegar
- 1 teaspoon dry mustard
- 1 teaspoon Worcestershire sauce
- 1 teaspoon anchovy paste
- ¼ cup extra-virgin olive oil
- ⅓ cup grated parmesan cheese
- Whole-wheat croutons (optional)

Directions:

1. In a large salad bowl, whisk together the garlic, sea salt, oil, lemon juice, vinegar, mustard, Worcestershire sauce, and anchovy paste.
2. Add lettuce and toss to evenly coat.
3. Sprinkle with the parmesan cheese.
4. Add whole-wheat croutons.

Marinated Veggie Stir-fry with Brown Rice

Ingredients:

- 1 large onion, cut into small slices
- 4 medium carrots, cut into small slices
- 2 medium zucchini, cut into small slices
- 2 large red peppers, cut into small pieces
- 2 medium yellow summer squash, cut into small pieces
- 3 tablespoons extra-virgin olive oil
- ¼ cup balsamic vinegar
- 1 teaspoon oregano, chopped

- 1 garlic clove, minced
- ¼ teaspoon sea salt
- ⅓ teaspoon ground coriander
- ¼ teaspoon ground cumin
- ⅓ teaspoon ground black pepper
- 1 teaspoon agave syrup
- 2 cups of cooked brown rice

Directions:

1. In a large bowl, combine 1 tablespoon oil, vinegar, oregano, garlic, coriander, cumin, sea salt, pepper, and agave syrup.
2. Add all the veggies and let stand for 30 minutes.
3. Drain the veggies and save the marinade.
4. In large skillet, heat the remaining 2 tablespoons of oil.
5. Cook the onion and carrots, stirring constantly for about 5 to 7 minutes.
6. Add the zucchini and squash, stirring constantly for another 2 to 3 minutes
7. Add the bell peppers and cook for another minute, stirring constantly.
8. Add 2 to 3 tablespoons of remaining marinade to the veggies and stir constantly until the veggies and marinade are hot, about 1 to 2 minutes more.
9. Serve over brown rice, if desired.

Cinnamon Granola

Ingredients:

- 3 cups rolled oats
- 2 teaspoons cinnamon
- ¼ cup agave nectar
- ½ cup chopped walnuts
- ½ cup unsweetened apple sauce

Directions:

1. Preheat oven to 325° F.
2. Put your grains and walnuts in a bowl and mix; then put in all remaining ingredients and whisk them.
3. Pour applesauce and agave nectar into the bowl with grains and blend well until it coats evenly.
4. Spread over a parchment-lined baking sheet and bake for 45 to 60 minutes, stirring every 10 to 15 minutes so it doesn't burn.
5. When it feels dry and has a golden brown color, it is ready. Cool before serving.

Cucumber Tomato Salad

Ingredients:

- 5 cups of heirloom tomatoes
- 2 small cucumbers
- 1 avocado, peeled and pitted
- ¼ red onion, finely chopped
- ¼ cup fresh basil, chopped

- 1 tablespoon red wine vinegar

- 2 tablespoons extra-virgin olive oil

Directions:

1. Chop tomatoes, cucumbers, and avocado into small, bite-size pieces and combine into a serving dish.

2. In separate bowl, combine onion, basil, vinegar, oil, and salt and pepper to taste.

3. Pour over tomatoes and serve.

Braised Tofu

Ingredients:

- 1 pound extra-firm tofu

- ¼ cup water

- 2 cloves garlic, minced

- 3 tablespoons fresh lemon juice

- 2 tablespoons soy sauce

- Olive oil cooking spray

Directions:

1. Turn oven to broil.

2. Press tofu (you do not have to squeeze it, just press some of the moisture out of it).

3. Cut tofu into triangles (makes about 16 triangles).

4. Mix all other ingredients (except tofu) in small bowl.

5. Spray olive oil on an oven pan or baking sheet

and dip each piece of tofu in the braising sauce and place on the pan/baking sheet.

6. Put the pan or baking sheet in the oven and bake for 10 minutes until tofu is lightly browned.

7. Remove the pan and pour a few spoonfuls of braising sauce over the tofu and put back in oven for 3 more minutes. Repeat one more time until tofu is golden brown. Remove from the oven and serve.

Sweet Potato Fries

Ingredients:

- 1 teaspoon chopped, fresh rosemary leaves

- 1 tablespoon extra-virgin olive oil

- 3 medium sweet potatoes

- ¼ teaspoon sea salt

Directions:

1. Preheat oven to 425° F.

2. In a small bowl, combine rosemary and olive oil and set aside.

3. Scrub potatoes and cut each potato lengthwise into ½ inch slices. Stacking 2 slices together, cut each into ½ inch strips.

4. In a large bowl, toss sweet potato strips with rosemary mixture until evenly coated.

5. Spread sweet potatoes on a large parchment-lined baking sheet in a single layer.

6. Bake for 30 to 35 minutes, flipping potatoes over halfway through baking time, until lightly browned.

7. Remove from oven, sprinkle with a little salt, and serve warm.

Collard Green Stew with Black-Eyed Peas

Ingredients:

- 8 cups of collard greens, cleaned and chopped
- 1 can cooked black-eyed peas, rinsed and drained
- 1 can no-sodium diced tomatoes
- 4 cups low-sodium vegetable broth
- Ground black pepper, to taste

Directions:

1. Bring broth and 2 cups water to a boil in a large saucepan on high heat.

2. Add collard greens, cover, and simmer for 15 minutes.

3. Add tomatoes and return to a simmer.

4. Cover and cook until tomatoes are tender.

5. Stir in black-eyed peas and simmer until heated through, about 2 minutes.

6. Season with pepper, to taste, and serve immediately.

Glossary

Calorie:

Calories are units of energy that fuel our bodies, just as gasoline fuels our cars. We get calories from the food we eat. When we consume food, our body breaks down this food and turns it into energy. A more scientific definition states it as the quantity of energy required to raise the temperature of one gram of water by one degree Celsius under standard conditions.

Carbohydrates (Carbs):

Carbohydrates, particularly those found in their natural form, contain most of the essential nutrients that keep you healthy, give you energy, and turn up your metabolism. Examples include fruit, vegetables, whole grains, beans, nuts, and seeds.

There are two main types of carbohydrates:

- *Complex carbs* are found in vegetables, nuts, fruits, seeds, and grains and include starch and dietary fiber. They take longer for the body to break down than simple carbs, which helps the body maintain a steady blood sugar level.

- *Refined carbs* (also known as simple carbs or sugars) are fruits, vegetables, or grains that have been processed away from their natural state, such as bleached white flour. Most of the vitamins and minerals have been processed out of refined carbs.

319

Fiber:

A compound found in plant-based foods. Fiber, sometimes called bulk or roughage, is the non-digestible portion of fruits, vegetables, and grains. There are two types of fiber:

- *Soluble fiber* dissolves and breaks down in water, forming a thick gel. Some food sources of soluble fiber include apples, oranges, peaches, nuts, barley, beets, carrots, cranberries, lentils, oats, bran, and peas. Soluble fiber slows the absorption of food after meals and thus helps regulate blood sugar and insulin levels, reducing fat storage in the body. It also removes unwanted toxins, lowers cholesterol, and reduces the risk of heart disease and gallstones.

- *Insoluble fiber* (also known as roughage) does not dissolve in water or break down in your digestive system. Insoluble fiber passes through the gastrointestinal tract almost intact. Some food sources of insoluble fiber include green leafy vegetables, seeds and nuts, fruit skins, potato skins, vegetable skins, wheat bran, and whole grains. Insoluble fiber not only promotes weight loss and relieves constipation, but it also assists in the removal of cancer-causing substances from the colon wall. It helps to prevent the formation of gallstones by binding with bile acids and removing cholesterol before stones can form, thus they are especially beneficial to people with diabetes or colon cancer.

Green Drink:

A nickname for a drink that is derived primarily from green leafy vegetables. A green drink is high in fiber, rich in vitamins, and low in calories. Green drinks help you detoxify and cleanse your system, lose weight, have more energy, and make the body more alkaline. When you drink them, the nutrients in them get to the cells very quickly and give the body a real boost.

Proteins:

Proteins are required for the structure, function, and regulation of the body's cells, tissues, and organs. Proteins are made up of amino acids that carry out unique functions and provide essential components for the muscles, skin, bones, and body as a whole. Sources of protein include beans, eggs, nuts, seeds, lean poultry, beef, fish, and seafood. Consuming enough protein helps you preserve lean muscle mass, and the more lean muscle you have, the more calories you burn, even at rest. Eating protein balances your blood sugar levels so you don't get spikes in energy throughout the day.

Sugar:

Also known as refined sugar, sugar goes through a process of "refining" to extract the sucrose (sugar) from the plant materials. Refined sugars are absorbed quickly upon consumption and contribute to a number of diseases and health risks. Although refined sugar is thought to be basic table sugar, there are actually a number of different types of refined sugars, which include high fructose corn syrup, dextrose (corn sugar), maltose (malt sugar), lactose (milk sugar), corn sweetener, raw sugar, brown sugar, powdered sugar, and molasses.

Toxins:

Any substance that irritates or creates harmful effects in the body or mind. Toxins are everywhere, and we are unknowingly filling our bodies with them every day. There are two types of toxins: environmental toxins and internal toxins.

- *Environmental toxins* are found outside the body/mind and include pollutants, smog, medications, hormones/birth control pills, medications, household cleaners, food additives, and pesticides.

- *Internal toxins* are found inside the body/mind and include bacterial/yeast/fungal overgrowth, parasite infections, chronic worry or fear, food allergies, and dental or medical implants, such as implants from cosmetic surgeries, joint replacements, or mercury dental fillings.

Bibliography

Bach, Peter B. (2010). "Postmenopausal Hormone Therapy and Breast Cancer." *JAMA*. 304(15):1719–1720.

Baillie-Hamilton, Paula F. (2002). "Chemical Toxins: A Hypothesis to Explain the Global Obesity Epidemic." *The Journal of Alternative and Complementary Medicine*, 8(2).

Bonds, Denise E., Zaccaro, Daniel J., Karter, Andrew J., Selby, Joe V, Saad, Mohammed, and Goff, Jr. David C. (2009). "Ethnic and Racial Differences in Diabetes Care: The Insulin Resistance Atherosclerosis Study." *Wake Forest University School of Medicine*, Medical Center Boulevard, Winston-Salem.

Braun, Barry. "Low intensity ambulation." *American College of Sports Medicine newsletter*.

Burroughs, Stanley. (1976). *The Master Cleanser: With Special Needs and Problems*. Reno, NV: Bourroughs Books.

Church, Timothy S., Earnest, Conrad P., Skinner, James S, and Blair, Steven. (2007). "Effects of Different Doses of Physical Activity on Cardiorespiratory Fitness Among Sedentary, Overweight or Obese Postmenopausal Women With Elevated Blood Pressure." *JAMA*. 297(19):2081–2091.

Cloud, John. (2009, August). "Why Exercise Won't Make You Thin." *Time*.

2>ght Without Dieting or Working Out!

Glickman, Peter, and Garcia, Carlos. (2011). *Lose Weight, Have More Energy and Be Happier in 10 Days: Take Charge of Your Health with the Master Cleanse*: Clearwater, Florida: Published by Peter Glickman.

Hill, James O. et. al. (2003). "Obesity and the Environment: Where Do We Go from Here?" Science. 299(5608):853–855.

Holford, Patrick, and Joyce, Fiona McDonald. (2010). *The 9-Day Liver Detox Diet: The Definitive Diet that Delivers Results.* New York: Crown Publishing Group.

Imbeault, P. (2002). "Weight-Loss induced in plasma pollutant is associated with reduced skeletal muscle oxidative capacity." *American Journal of Physiology-Endocrinology and Metabolism.* 282(3):E574–79.

Katzmarzyk, Peter T. (2011). "Black women can carry more weight than white women and still be considered healthy." *Reuters Health.*

Kendrick, Alex, and Kendrick, Stephen. (2008). *The Love Dare.* Tennessee: B&H Books.

Koh-Banerjee. (2004). "Whole grains and less weight gain." P. *American Journal of Clinical Nutrition*, 80:1237–1245.

Kuk, Jennifer L., Katzmarzyk, Peter T. Nichaman, Milton Z., Church, Timothy S., Blair, Steven N., Ross, Robert. (2006). "Visceral Fat Is an Independent Predictor of All-cause Mortality in Men." *Obesity.*

Lee, Dr. John, and Hopkins, Virginia. (2006). *Dr. John Lee's Hormone Balance Made Simple: The Essential How-to Guide to Symptoms, Dosage, Timing, and More*. New York: Grand Central Life & Style.

Lenoir, M., Serre, F., Cantin, L., and Ahmed, S.H. (2007). "Intense sweetness surpasses cocaine reward." PLoS ONE 2: e698.

Ogden, C., Fryar, C., Carroll, M., and Flegal, K. (2004). Mean body weight, height, and body mass index in the United States, 1960–2002: Advanced Data from Vital and Health Statistics. *National Center for Health Statistics*.

Pelletier, C. (2002). "Toxicological Sciences: Associations between weight-loss induced changes in plasma organochlorine concentrations, serum t3 concentration, and resting metabolic rate."

Pestic, Monit J. (1986). Environmental Protection Agency National Human Adipose Tissue Survey. Sep 6 (2):84–88. *National Human Adipose Tissue Survey Specimens Volume III*.

Platt, Michael B. (2007). *The Miracle of Bio-Identical Hormones*. California: Claney Lane Publishing.

Rahman, Mahbubur, and Berenson, Abbey. (2010). Accuracy of current body mass index obesity classification for white, black and Hispanic reproductive-age women. *Obstet Gynecol*. 115(5): 982–988.

Robinson, Jo. *Why Grassfed Is Best!: The Surprising Benefits of Grassfed Meats, Eggs, and Dairy Products*. Washington: Vashon Island Press, 2000.

Somers, Suzanne. *Ageless: The Naked Truth About Bioidentical Hormones*. (2006). New York: Crown Publishing Group.

Somers, Suzanne, and Greene, Robert A. (2005). *The Sexy Years: Discover the Hormone Connection: The Secret to Fabulous Sex, Great Health, and Vitality for Women and Men*. New York: Crown Publishers.

Watson, Brenda. (2007). *The Fiber35 Diet: Nature's Weight Loss Secret*. New York: Free Press.

Wurtman, R.J., and Wurtman, J. (1995). "Brand serotonin, carbohydrates, obesity, and depression." *Obesity Research* 4: 477S–480S.

About the Author

JJ Smith is a nutritionist and certified weight-loss expert, passionate relationship/life coach, and inspirational speaker. She has been featured on *The Steve Harvey Show*, *The Montel Williams Show*, *The Jamie Foxx Show*, and *The Michael Baisden Show*. JJ has made appearances on the NBC, FOX, CBS, and CW Network television stations, as well as in the pages of *Glamour*, *Essence*, *Heart and Soul*, and *Ladies Home Journal*. Since reclaiming her health, losing weight, and discovering a "second youth" in her forties, bestselling author JJ Smith has become the voice of inspiration to those who want to lose weight, be healthy, and get their sexy back! JJ Smith provides lifestyle solutions for losing weight, getting healthy, looking younger, and improving your love life! To learn more, check out www.jjsmithonline.com.

JJ has dedicated her life to the field of healthy eating and living. JJ's passion is to educate others and share with them the natural remedies to stay slim, restore health, and look and feel younger. JJ has studied many philosophies of natural healing and learned from some of the great teachers of our time. After studying and applying knowledge about how to heal the body and lose weight, JJ went on to receive several certifications—one as a certified nutritionist and another as a certified weight-management expert. JJ received her certification as a nutritionist from the International Institute of Holistic Healing. She received her certification as a weight-management specialist from the National Exercise and Sports Trainers Association (NESTA). She is also a member of the American Nutrition Association (ANA).

JJ is also the author of the bestseller *Why I Love Men: The Joys of Dating*. It contains compelling and funny stories she cultivated over the past fifteen years of relationships that included three marriage proposals. In a sister-to-sister, woman-to-woman approach, JJ shares her heartfelt story of her joys, pains, and lessons learned from dating. She also provides scores of tips on how women can improve their relationships with men and have more fun while dating. *Why I Love Men* is ultimately a tribute to men and how they shaped her life and helped her grow and develop as a woman.

JJ holds a B.A. in mathematics from Hampton University in Virginia. She continued her education by completing The Wharton Business School Executive Management Certificate program. She currently serves as vice president and partner in an IT consulting firm, Intact Technology, Inc., in Greenbelt, Maryland. JJ was also the youngest African American to receive a vice president position at a Fortune 500 company. Her hobbies include reading, writing, and deejaying.

Acknowledgments

M om and Dad, thanks for giving me every opportunity to succeed in life. The two of you have given me wisdom, strength, and encouragement, and you made me know God when I was little, whether I wanted to or not. Mom, you provide me with a model of a beautiful queen every day. Don't ever change!

Todd, my best friend, whom I love so dearly. No one outside of my family has loved me as much as you do. If you get one great love in a lifetime, for me, you are it!

To my brothers, Jay and Johnny, and my cousin, Troy, thanks for loving and protecting me throughout my life. Jay, thanks especially for always encouraging me in everything I do; you have always supported and encouraged me, and never judged me...and I have had some crazy a#!& ideas!

To my uncles—Thomas, Edward, and Spencer—all of you showed me what it is to provide for and take care of a family.

To my aunts—Elsie, Aggie, Sandy, Maggie, Connie, Theresa, and Judy—all of you showed me how to love and care for a man. Both my aunts and uncles have shown me love since the day I was born.

To my cousins, who grew up with me like sisters— Karen, Tina, Vickie, Darlene, Tiffany, Lashanda, Rhonda, Cheryl, and Cassandra. Some of my most memorable times in life have been with all of you. Thanks to all of my other cousins and two very special cousins, Kenny and Kathy, who have loved, supported, and encouraged me all my life.

To "The Fellas" who make every day at work fun and enjoyable: Eric B., Mike C., Russ B., Jesse K., and Bruce T. Thank you for your friendship. You all thoroughly entertain and care for me each and every day. You are truly my extended family for life.

To my best girlfriend, Bridget. You have made life's journey over the years fun and enjoyable. Every part of my life has been influenced and made better by you.

To my entire Intact family—I'm fortunate to have had the opportunity to work with some of the smartest people that I have ever met in my lifetime—Todd, Jesse, Derek, Sherrie, Brandon, and all the other Intact team members.

Thanks to my thoughtful, talented editor, Carrie Cantor, who went above and beyond and constantly exceeded my expectations. My appreciation also goes to my gifted book cover and interior designer, Irene Archer. To Roy Cox, my incredible photographer, who just didn't take photos of me but made me feel like a supermodel. Thanks for making the photo shoot a memorable experience.

To the women that I have never met who inspire me each and every day—Oprah Winfrey, Michelle Obama, and Hillary Clinton.

And, last but not least, thanks to my Lord and Savior, Jesus Christ, for giving me an abundant life!